Blue Marble Health

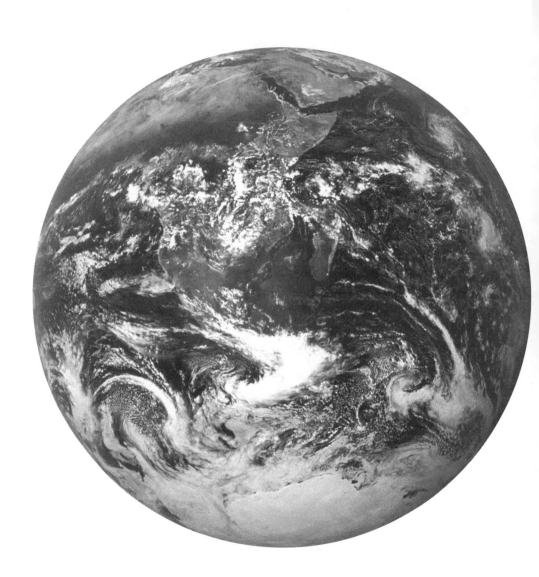

Blue Marble Health

An Innovative Plan to Fight Diseases of the Poor amid Wealth

Peter J. Hotez, MD, PhD

Baylor College of Medicine

Johns Hopkins University Press

Baltimore

Johns Hopkins University Press
2715 North Charles Street
Baltimore, Maryland 21218-4363
www.press.jhu.edu

Library of Congress Cataloging-in-Publication Data

Names: Hotez, Peter J., author
Title: Blue marble health : an innovative plan to fight diseases of the poor amid wealth /
Peter J. Hotez ; with a foreword by Cher.
Description: Baltimore : Johns Hopkins University Press, 2016. | Includes
    bibliographical references and index.
Identifiers: LCCN 2015046697| ISBN 9781421420462 (pbk. : alk. paper) | ISBN
    1421420465 (pbk. : alk. paper) | ISBN 9781421420479 (electronic) | ISBN
    1421420473 (electronic)
Subjects: | MESH: Neglected Diseases—economics | Poverty Areas | Global
    Health—economics | Health Equity—economics | Tropical Medicine—economics
Classification: LCC RA418.5.P6 | NLM W 74.1 | DDC 362.1086/942—dc23
    LC record available at http://lccn.loc.gov/2015046697

A catalog record for this book is available from the British Library.

The quotation from John Lennon on the facing page has been ascribed to Allen Saunders,
who wrote in *Reader's Digest* in the 1950s, "Life is what happens to us while we are making
other plans" (http://www.huffingtonpost.com/claudia-gryvatz-copquin/gilda-radner_b
_2231040.html).

*Special discounts are available for bulk purchases of this book. For more information, please
contact Special Sales at 410-516-6936 or specialsales@press.jhu.edu.*

Johns Hopkins University Press uses environmentally friendly book materials, including
recycled text paper that is composed of at least 30 percent post-consumer waste,
whenever possible.

To my champions and mentors in Texas:

Mark Kline, MD, and Mark Wallace of Texas Children's Hospital

Paul Klotman, MD, President of Baylor College of Medicine

Amb. Edward P. Djerejian, Director, James A. Baker III Institute for Public Policy, Rice University

Philip K. Russell, MD, President Emeritus, Sabin Vaccine Institute

And to my wife, Ann Hotez, and our four children, Matthew, Emily, Daniel, and our (now adult) special needs daughter, Rachel Hotez, who helps to keep me humble and reminds me daily of what John Lennon once wrote and sang:

"Life is what happens while you are busy making other plans."

Contents

Foreword

During more than five decades as an artist and performer on the world stage, I have been extremely blessed to visit dozens of nations and meet tens of thousands of amazing people of all religions and ethnic backgrounds. Connecting with people from all walks of life has been an energizing life force and an inspiration for my work. But I have also witnessed a dark side to our big and beautiful planet, namely, the dehumanizing effects of severe poverty. For me, there is nothing more devastating than seeing parents who cannot afford to care for or feed their children or seeing the desperate homeless.

In response, I have tried to give back to those most in need. Through our Cher Charitable Foundation, we have helped the poorest people living in Armenia as well as children with craniofacial deformities, head and neck diseases, and neglected diseases such as pediatric AIDS and cerebral malaria. Most recently, through our support of the Peace Village School in Shikamana, Kenya, hundreds of orphans and other vulnerable children are getting a fresh start. We are beginning to make a difference.

Aside from the challenges of being poor, it must also be especially disheartening to be poor and to live alongside great wealth. It's a terrible thing to live as a "have not" next to a "have." Yet in communities across America, more than one million families must survive on practically no money and barely scratch out an existence. These same destitute families usually live within a few miles or even a few blocks from those with enormous wealth and privilege.

Now, with the latest findings of Dr. Peter Hotez, we realize there's a new dimension to extreme poverty. In the United States, or indeed anywhere

where wealthy people live, including Europe, Australia, Southeast Asia, and Central and South America, Peter finds an astonishing but mostly hidden level of poverty and suffering. He has discovered that most of the poverty-related diseases, sometimes known as the neglected tropical diseases, or NTDs, actually occur in the wealthiest countries and economies. Our old concept of global health—developed versus less developed countries–is morphing. In its place, the NTDs are abundant wherever you find hardship. We now learn that it doesn't matter much if that poverty is in Lagos, Luanda, Lahore, La Paz, or Los Angeles. Peter's framework, which he names "blue marble health," means that the NTDs will be found regardless of location as long as there are places or regions where people live in desperate circumstances. Blue marble health has important implications for both global public health and public policy. Peter finds that if the elected leaders of the most powerful nations would simply recognize and support their own impoverished and neglected populations, a majority of our most ancient and terrible scourges could vanish.

I hope this book is an inspiration to young people thinking about a future career in the sciences, the humanities, or in the health professions. I also hope that the concept of blue marble health will inspire our global leaders to take charge of their own vulnerable populations who have neglected diseases. Currently, more than a billion people live with no money and suffer from horrific NTDs. The fact that they are mostly hidden away and forgotten in wealthy countries is inexcusable. This must be fixed.

Cher
Malibu, California

Preface

In 2006, I became the founding editor in chief of *PLOS Neglected Tropical Diseases*, a then new journal for a growing community of scientists and public health experts committed to studying the neglected tropical diseases (NTDs). As part of the Public Library of Science, *PLOS Neglected Tropical Diseases* was the first open access journal exclusively devoted to NTDs. A few years ago, I was joined by Yale University's Dr. Serap Aksoy as co-editor in chief, together with a distinguished group of deputy editors and associate editors working all over the world. We have benefited from the able guidance of the PLOS staff based in San Francisco, including Jeri Wright, Alicia Zuniga, Catherine Nancarrow, and Dr. Larry Peiperl.

One of the surprises about our journal over this past decade has been the number of papers we received from scientists in middle-income countries, especially the BRICS—Brazil, Russia, India, China, and South Africa. Moreover, the papers discussed findings from studies that went beyond the poorest and most destitute nations in the world. I became deeply impressed with the number of papers reporting on disease findings in middle-income countries, and even in some high-income countries. This observation, combined with my personal experiences after moving to Texas and seeing firsthand the endemic neglected tropical diseases, inspired me to look more deeply into the problem of the health disparities of the poor who live in the midst of wealth. I first wrote about the concept of "blue marble health" in both *Foreign Policy* and *PLOS Neglected Tropical Diseases* in 2013, with subsequent articles in 2015. Nathaniel Gore, together with Dr. Peiperl, also created two *PLOS* collections of articles devoted to blue marble health.

Many of the findings in this book are based on data and information published in *PLOS Neglected Tropical Diseases* by a wide range of investigators. These articles are cited in the text and then listed by chapter at the end of the book. Another important source of data is the Preventive Chemotherapy and Transmission Control Databank of the World Health Organization and its Department of Neglected Tropical Diseases, previously headed by my friend and colleague Dr. Lorenzo Savioli, and now under the direction of Dr. Dirk Engels. Also essential for our findings on blue marble health are data from the Global Burden of Disease Study led by Dr. Christopher J. L. Murray, who heads the Institute for Health Metrics and Evaluation at the University of Washington in Seattle.

My colleagues at the Department of State and White House and their US Science Envoy program also provided a fresh perspective on the geopolitics of diseases and science and health diplomacy. They included Undersecretary Catherine Novelli, White House Science Advisor Dr. John Holdren, Assistant Secretary Judith Garber, Deputy Assistant Secretary Dr. Jonathan Margolis, Dr. Bruce Ruscio, Dr. Matthew West, Kimberly Coleman, Stephanie Hutchison, Kay Hairston, Daisy Dix, Amani Mekki, Patricia Hill, Douglas Apostol, Christopher Rich, and Kia Henry. Prof. Neal Lane at Rice University's Baker Institute has also been an important mentor.

I also want to thank our many donors and partners who make it possible for us to develop new vaccines and other innovations for neglected diseases among the poor. The Bill & Melinda Gates Foundation, the National Institute of Allergy and Infectious Diseases, and the Fogarty International Center of the National Institutes of Health got us started, while today our new partners include Texas Children's Hospital, the Carlos Slim Foundation, the Kleberg Foundation, Dr. Gary Michelson and the Michelson Medical Research Foundation, Len Benkenstein and the Southwest Electronic Energy Medical Research Institute, the Dutch government and its Ministry of Foreign Affairs, the European Union and the Amsterdam Institute of Global Health and Development, the Brazilian Ministry of Health, and the Japanese GHIT Fund.

I am especially grateful to Nathaniel Wolf, who helps me on editorial matters at the National School of Tropical Medicine at Baylor College of Medicine. In addition to being a great sounding board and adviser on editorial issues, Nathaniel took on the important role of obtaining permissions for reproducing many of the figures for this book and working closely with our publisher. The photographer Anna Grove also contributed unique pictures of Houston's Fifth Ward. I also want to thank Dr. Jennifer Herricks, my first and only postdoctoral fellow in public policy, for helping me to create and shape the "worm index" of human development, and Vernesta Jackson, my assistant, for helping to keep me organized. Dr. Maria Elena Bottazzi is the deputy director of the Sabin Vaccine Institute product development partnership and the associate dean of the National School of Tropical Medicine at Baylor College of Medicine. Her leadership and organizational abilities made it possible for me to have the freedom to think creatively and write.

My wife, Ann Hotez, provided incredible support to make it possible for me to write a book, as did my four children—Matthew, Emily, Rachel, and Daniel. I would also like to thank Agora (once voted "best coffeehouse" by the Houston Press), which is located in my neighborhood of Montrose, as well as the Hotel Galvez, located in Galveston, Texas, for providing good escape venues in which to write when I needed them.

Finally, I want to thank my publisher, Johns Hopkins University Press, and its editor for public health and health policy, Robin W. Coleman, for their helpful and timely editorial advice and activities.

Blue Marble Health

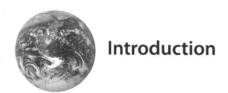

Introduction

In 2011, together with a team of 15 scientists, I relocated to Houston, Texas, to launch a new school devoted to poverty-related diseases. The National School of Tropical Medicine at Baylor College of Medicine is a joint venture among three biomedical institutions—Baylor, Texas Children's Hospital, and the Sabin Vaccine Institute—with a mission devoted to research on and training in the treatment of neglected tropical diseases, or NTDs (see box I.1). Today, the NTDs represent the most common afflictions of people who live in extreme poverty. These ailments include parasitic diseases such as hookworm, schistosomiasis, Chagas disease, and leishmaniasis—or, as I often say, the most important diseases you've never heard of. Virtually every impoverished individual is infected with at least one NTD.

An unusual aspect of Baylor's National School of Tropical Medicine is that it includes as its research arm a unique type of organization known as a product development partnership (PDP). There are 16 PDPs worldwide. They are international nonprofit organizations that develop and manufacture biopharmaceuticals—drugs, diagnostics, and vaccines—for the NTDs, as well as for HIV/AIDS, tuberculosis (TB), and malaria. Together, the NTDs and AIDS, TB, and malaria are sometimes broadly defined as "neglected diseases." PDPs develop and test new products for neglected diseases that the major pharmaceutical companies may not have an interest in because they are poverty-related afflictions that will therefore not generate significant sales income. The National School of Tropical Medicine's PDP is known as the Sabin Vaccine Institute PDP, and it is specifically focused on developing NTD vaccines.

Box I.1.
The Poverty-Related Diseases: Neglected Tropical Diseases (NTDs) and Other Neglected Diseases

NTDs: The neglected tropical diseases are a group of chronic and debilitating poverty-related illnesses. Most, but not all, are parasitic diseases. An original list of 13 NTDs published in *PLOS Medicine* in 2005 has since been expanded by the World Health Organization to include 17 major conditions:

> Soil-transmitted helminth infections (including ascariasis, trichuriasis, hookworm infection, strongyloidiasis, and toxocariasis)
> Lymphatic filariasis (elephantiasis)
> Dracunculiasis (guinea worm disease)
> Onchocerciasis (river blindness)
> Schistosomiasis
> Foodborne trematodiases
> Taeniasis and neurocysticercosis
> Echinococcosis
> Human African trypanosomiasis (sleeping sickness)
> Chagas disease (American trypanosomiasis)
> Leishmaniasis
> Yaws
> Buruli ulcer
> Trachoma
> Leprosy
> Rabies
> Dengue and other arboviral infections

PLOS Neglected Tropical Diseases has published a further expanded list that also includes several intestinal protozoan infections, chronic fungal infections, cholera and other bacterial diseases, and ectoparasitic infections such as scabies and myiasis. Types of malaria other than those caused by *Plasmodium falciparum* (such as *Plasmodium vivax*) are also sometimes considered to be NTDs.

Neglected Diseases: There are several different definitions of neglected diseases. Here I refer to neglected diseases as NTDs together with the "big three" diseases—HIV/AIDS, malaria, and tuberculosis. A similar usage has been adopted by the G-FINDER report on research funding for neglected diseases. There are several reasons that the term "neglected" is used for both groups of conditions, including (1) lack of attention by government leaders and international agencies; (2) the strong links of these diseases to vulnerable populations and to people who live in extreme poverty and are thus often hidden or ignored; and (3) low levels of research funding and support.

One reason I was so eager to move our scientists to Houston was to take advantage of being located within the Texas Medical Center. The TMC is more than just the world's largest medical center; it is a medical city comprising more than 50 biomedical institutions and 100,000 employees, occupying building space that exceeds that of downtown Los Angeles. A second reason for the relocation was the generous support we received from Texas Children's Hospital (the world's largest children's hospital), which also housed the Sabin Vaccine Institute PDP in a modern research building known as the Feigin Center, named for the late Ralph Feigin, MD, one of the giants in the treatment of pediatric infectious diseases. Our goal for moving and becoming linked to the TMC was to increase the number of new vaccines we are creating for the poorest people in less developed countries, as well as to accelerate the pace at which they are produced. It was an amazing opportunity to leverage the facilities of more than 50 world-class institutions in order to launch an assault on global poverty-related diseases. The laboratories began operations in the fall of 2011, and today we have two vaccines in clinical trials—for human hookworm infection and schistosomiasis—with others in various stages of product development.

PDPs are nonprofit product development partnerships committed to developing new products for neglected diseases.

Within a few months after moving to Houston, we learned about a different side of the city. Driving just a few miles from the TMC, I began to see a level of extreme poverty that I had not previously imagined existed in the continental United States. A stark example of the severe impoverishment found in Houston (and elsewhere in Texas) is an area known as the Fifth Ward (fig. I.1), a political division of Houston located northeast of the downtown area. Following the American Civil War, freed slaves settled in this area, and today the Fifth Ward represents one of several important African American communities in the city. Driving my car deep into this neighborhood reminded me of the terrible poverty I had seen as a scientist investigating tropical diseases in destitute areas of Honduras, Guatemala, Brazil, and China. I saw abandoned buildings, dilapidated housing with no window screens, uncollected garbage, clogged drainage ditches that smelled like sewage, discarded tires filled with water, and packs of stray and roaming dogs. I thought to myself, these images look just like the standard global disease movie typically shown to first-year public health or medical students. A little bit of Lagos (Nigeria's largest city) right here in Texas.

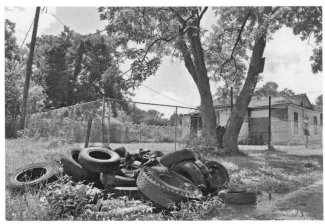

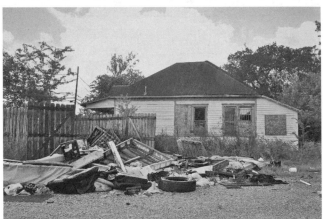

Figure I.1.
Houston's historic Fifth Ward: dilapidated housing, discarded tires, and piles of garbage. Photos by Anna Grove.

It was even more astonishing when we turned our global health lens inward to study diseases that were affecting impoverished areas such as the Fifth Ward. Without looking very hard, we found widespread NTDs among the poor living in Texas and elsewhere in the southern United States. It struck me that although we designate these diseases as "tropical," the NTDs are first and foremost diseases of acute poverty. Ultimately, we determined that 12 million Americans who live at such poverty levels suffer from at least one NTD. The diseases include neglected parasitic infections such as Chagas disease, cysticercosis, toxocariasis, and trichomoniasis [1].

The finding of widespread NTDs among the poor living in the United States was eye opening and caused me to delve deeper into the problem of poverty-related illnesses in wealthy countries. We found that most of the world's neglected diseases—including the NTDs and, to some extent, HIV/AIDS, tuberculosis, and malaria, as well as some important noncommunicable diseases—can be found among the poor who live amidst wealth. Thus, the traditional concept of global health that compares unique diseases in less developed countries (especially in sub-Saharan Africa) with more developed countries (such as the United States and countries in western Europe) no longer applied. With the exception of a few countries devastated by armed conflict, almost all national economies are on the rise, but they are leaving behind a bottom segment of society that still suffers from the NTDs and other neglected diseases. Startlingly, I have determined that, in addition to Nigeria, most of the world's neglected diseases are actually also found in the wealthiest economies, including the Group of 20 (G20) nations. Unraveling some of the details around this observation is a key goal of this book.

That most of the world's neglected diseases are highly prevalent in G20 economies has important public health and policy implications. Because I believe that widespread poverty-related diseases in wealthy countries represent a paradigm shift from traditional notions of global health, I have given this framework a new name: "blue marble health." This commemorates the amazing images of planet Earth that the Apollo 17 astronauts first photographed as they orbited the moon in 1972 [2]. The "blue marble" became an important symbol of peace and healing [3], and it is a fitting metaphor for the pursuit of worldwide good health and efforts to alleviate human suffering from the devastating ailments associated with indigence in all nations.

Blue marble health refers to a changing global health paradigm in which the world's neglected diseases and NTDs are increasingly found among the extremely poor who live amidst wealth. The concept of the blue marble refers to an iconic picture of Earth taken by the Apollo 17 astronauts and now considered a symbol of peace and healing. Ultimately, blue marble health provides a new framework for shaping public policy to control or eliminate some of the world's worst poverty-related illnesses.

A Changing Landscape in Global Health

Encountering poor people and diseases of the poor in proximity to wealth is not new, but it is remarkable that these populations account for so much of today's global burden of neglected diseases. A key force driving blue marble health and the finding that most of the world's neglected diseases now occur in wealthy nations may be related to substantial success over the past 15 years in reducing those diseases in the world's most devastated low-income countries, especially in Africa. As the incidence and prevalence of these neglected diseases began to diminish, a new health landscape was revealed.

Has peeling the onion exposed a new paradigm? In 2000, the attention of the then Group of 8 (G8) countries (now G7 with the departure of the Russian Federation) turned to Africa and other profoundly impoverished regions. This notice was manifested under the auspices of a set of United Nations Millennium Development Goals (MDGs) that were developed to address global poverty. Described here are some amazing gains that were achieved in Africa and elsewhere by means of these goals. Before describing blue marble health in any further detail, let's first look at what happened between the years 2000 and 2015 in the world's poorest countries, notably in Africa.

Launched in 2000, the MDGs represent an ambitious set of eight goals (together with specific targets for each of the goals) that were established to sustain poverty reduction, particularly among the group sometimes known as the "bottom billion"—the more than one billion people who live below the World Bank poverty figure, then set at $1.25 per day, but recently increased to $1.90 per day (fig. 1.1). What impresses me most about the MDGs is how they

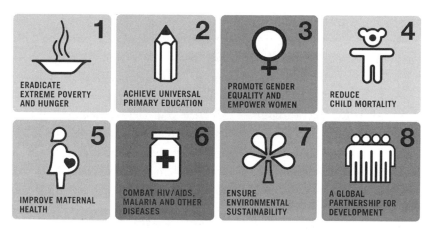

Figure 1.1.
The United Nations' Millennium Development Goals
(MDGs), 2000–2015. Courtesy of UNDP Brazil.

effectively provided a key policy framework for channeling overseas development assistance, especially for many of the infectious diseases found among
the poor. A rationale for linking infectious diseases to poverty arose in part
from landmark reports from the World Bank, including a 1993 World Development Report titled "Investing in Health," led by Dr. Dean Jamison and others; an international Commission on Macroeconomics and Health, led by the
development economist Dr. Jeffrey Sachs; and the Commission for Africa,
under the leadership of then British Prime Minister Tony Blair [1].

Ultimately, two of the MDGs that heavily emphasized infectious diseases of the poor—MDG 4 "to reduce child mortality" and MDG 6 "to combat AIDS, malaria, and other diseases"—stand out for how elected leaders
and heads of state came together in order to respond to a global health crisis, especially in sub-Saharan Africa [2]. In my opinion, the international
response to these two goals and its convergence on Africa represent the first
of the truly great humanitarian achievements of this new century.

One reason I am confident about the successes of MDGs 4 and 6 is because of an initiative by the Bill & Melinda Gates Foundation to specifically
measure the morbidity and mortality toll from each of the major human
diseases and to examine how that burden of disease has changed over the
past two decades. The Global Burden of Disease Study (GBD) actually
began in 1990, but it was relaunched in order to assess individual disease
burdens for the year 2010 (GBD 2010) and then again for 2013 (GBD 2013).

Led by Dr. Christopher J. L. Murray, who heads the Seattle-based Institute for Health Metrics at the University of Washington, the GBD 2010 and GBD 2013 brought together hundreds of investigators worldwide (including this author) to determine the impact of up to 300 different disease conditions (ranging from infectious diseases to noncommunicable ailments such as cancer, diabetes, and heart disease to injuries) [3]. The health impact of each condition is measured both in terms of annual deaths and disability. The disability component is especially important because many of the most common NTDs, such as hookworm infection and schistosomiasis, are major disablers, although they are not necessarily leading killers. Together, years of life lost (YLLs) and years lived with disability (YLDs) are combined to produce a metric known as the disability-adjusted life year (DALY).

The GAVI Alliance and MDG 4

An important action item inspired by MDG 4 "to reduce child mortality" was to create an alliance of partners committed to fighting childhood deaths that could be prevented through vaccination. The major approaches include the development and distribution of vaccines, together with expanded coverage for immunization, with more people vaccinated in more geographic areas than ever before. The global alliance of vaccines and immunization, now known as Gavi, The Vaccine Alliance, is an international organization based in Geneva that was specifically established in 2000 to introduce new and underused vaccines, such as those for *Haemophilus influenzae* type B (Hib) meningitis and respiratory hepatitis B, while promoting the development and dissemination of new vaccines for rotavirus infection and pneumococcal pneumonia and meningitis. In parallel, coverage for childhood vaccines against diphtheria, tetanus, whooping cough, polio, measles, and other infections was expanded. The impact of this approach, now being carried out under the umbrella of a Global Vaccine Action Plan (GVAP), has been remarkable.

Shown in table 1.1 are some of the results published by GBD 2013 that compare childhood deaths between 1990 and 2013 [3]. Overall, the results indicate more than 50% reductions in deaths from major childhood killer diseases. The study estimates that the number of children under the age of five who die annually from infectious and related diseases has dropped by more than one-half, from 6.0 million deaths in 1990 to almost 2.8 million deaths in 2013. Many of these gains can be ascribed to increased vaccine coverage, together with the introduction of new vaccines for rotavirus and pneumococcus.

These dramatic decreases in childhood deaths partly point to the power of vaccines. Such reductions also are important advocacy tools to persuade essential donors and partners, including the United States government and European parliaments, to support Gavi and the GVAP. I also believe that this information simultaneously helps to counter a highly vocal and sometimes aggressive antivaccine lobby in the United States, Europe, and now even some of the large middle-income countries. As a consequence of "anti-vaxer" activities in recent years, we have seen unprecedented measles outbreaks in the United States, the United Kingdom, and elsewhere, long after measles was declared eliminated in those countries. Recently, Heidi Larson and her colleagues at the London School of Hygiene and Tropical Medicine derived a new "vaccine hes-

Global childhood mortality has been cut in half. Many of these gains can be attributed to greater awareness of the opportunity to prevent childhood illness through the use of vaccines, together with the activities of Gavi to introduce new vaccines and enhanced efforts by the governments of the major disease-endemic countries to vaccinate children and expand coverage.

Table 1.1. Median percentage change in deaths from childhood killer diseases, 1990 to 2013

Disease	Median % change (all ages)	Median % change (children age 1–59 months)
Measles	−83.0	−83.1
Tetanus	−82.1	−91.2
Diphtheria	−57.7	Not reported
Whooping cough	−56.7	−57.1
Diarrheal disease (including rotavirus)	−51.0	−68.0
Haemophilus influenzae type b (Hib) meningitis	−45.4	−54.0[a]
Pneumococcal meningitis	−29.4	−54.0[a]

Source: [3], http://dx.doi.org/10.1016/S0140–6736(14)61682–2.
[a] Reported for meningitis only, etiology not specified.

itancy" index in order to rank countries according to their rates of vaccine use versus refusal to vaccinate [4].

For me it is a source of enormous frustration that even though study after study has convincingly refuted any links between vaccines and autism, this issue continues to come up in state legislatures across the United States, reflecting a worrisome trend and increasing numbers of parents who choose to opt out of vaccinating their children. I am particularly concerned about antivaccine sentiments in highly populated middle-income countries such as the BRICS nations—Brazil, Russia, India, China, and South Africa—and also in some of the large nations belonging to the Organisation of Islamic Cooperation (OIC) such as Bangladesh, Indonesia, Nigeria, and Pakistan, where diseases such as measles and pertussis are still commonly found [5]. Encouraging the resistance of parents to vaccination could reverse the gains seen in some of these countries over the past twenty years.

In addition to being an academic dean and vaccine researcher, I am also the father of four, including an adult child with autism and severe mental and developmental disabilities. Yet I am willing to state publicly the lack of any evidence linking vaccines and autism [6]. My view is based on what we know regarding the genetic and epigenetic basis of the autism spectrum disorders, and the fact that changes in the prefrontal cortex of the brain of a child with autism begin prior to birth and well before an infant receives his or her first vaccination [7]. I hope we can stop the export of vaccine hesitancy from the United States and Europe to the large middle-income countries. Otherwise, we could face a reversal of the gains in reducing childhood deaths since the launch of MDG 4 and Gavi.

PEPFAR, PMI, GFATM, and MDG 6

The GBD 2013 has also measured an important effect produced by major interventions related to MDG 6 "to combat AIDS, malaria, and other diseases." In the years immediately following the proclamation of the MDGs, the White House under the administration of President George W. Bush initiated two large-scale programs for HIV/AIDS and malaria [8]. The President's Emergency Plan for AIDS Relief (PEPFAR) was launched following the 2003 State of the Union address, with a goal to place people living with

HIV/AIDS in sub-Saharan Africa and other less developed countries on antiretroviral therapy, in addition to implementing other prevention measures. Initially $15 billion was authorized over five years (and then reauthorized in 2008) [8]. In 2005, President Bush also established the President's Malaria Initiative (PMI) for $1.2 billion over five years to deliver mosquito nets and drugs to treat malaria [8]. In parallel, in 2002, the G8 nations initiated a Global Fund to Fight AIDS, Tuberculosis, and Malaria (GFATM), with the United States becoming the largest contributor [8]. The impact of these massive initiatives linked to MDG 6 was assessed by the GBD 2013, and the results are almost as impressive as they are for MDG 4 [9].

Through PEPFAR, PMI, and GFATM, impressive gains have been achieved in reducing deaths from AIDS, TB, and malaria.

Briefly, by 2013, upward trends in both HIV/AIDS and malaria deaths were reversed. The number of HIV-related deaths decreased from 1.7 million to 1.3 million, and because of the widespread use of antiretroviral therapies, an estimated 19.1 million life years were saved [8, 9]. For malaria, both the number of cases and deaths dropped approximately 30%, from 232 million cases (peaking in 2003) and 1.2 million deaths (peaking in 2004) to 165 million cases and 0.85 million deaths in 2013 [8, 9]. There were also important reductions in the incidence of TB. Thus, while substantial sums were spent between 2000 and 2011, including more than $50 billion for HIV/AIDS, $10 billion for malaria, and $8 billion for tuberculosis [9], there is no question that overseas development assistance for these "big three" diseases had a substantial impact.

Ascendancy of the Noncommunicable Diseases (NCDs)

It appears that the world's poorest countries particularly benefited from many of these MDG 4 and 6 interventions, with some of the greatest gains seen in lowered mortality for certain childhood-preventable diseases, malaria, and HIV/AIDS in Africa. It is also apparent that the initiatives launched under the auspices of the MDGs are having huge and important effects and need to continue as we approach the year 2020 and beyond. However, paralleling these important reductions in deaths and DALYs from childhood vaccine-preventable diseases, AIDS, TB, and malaria, an emerging increase has been observed for many of the noncommunicable diseases (NCDs), especially those linked to high mortality such as cancer, cardiovascular diseases, chronic respiratory conditions, and diabetes.

The GBD 2010 noted that while the world's DALYs remained more or less fixed at around 2.5 billion between 1990 (2.502 billion) and 2010 (2.490 billion), the relative proportion of DALYs from communicable versus noncommunicable diseases shifted significantly over this period. Thus, the DALYs from communicable diseases, together with maternal, neonatal, and nutritional disorders, decreased by 26.5% over that twenty-year period, but there was a commensurate 25.0% rise in NCDs [10]. Included in those numbers was a whopping 37% increase in DALYs from mental and behavioral disorders, led by unipolar depressive disorders, and more than a 50% increase in DALYs from neurological disorders, including Alzheimer's disease (and other dementias) and epilepsy. There was also a 69% rise in the DALYs from diabetes mellitus [10].

The global decrease in deaths and DALYs from infectious diseases has been accompanied by a commensurate rise in NCDs.

The factors responsible for this rise in NCDs are multiple and include mounting tobacco use and air pollution, dietary and other lifestyle changes, urbanization and the stresses of urban living, and increases in alcohol and other substance abuse, among others. It is also possible that reductions in infectious diseases are allowing people to live longer and acquire NCDs. I think the reductions in infectious and communicable diseases at the expense of a rise in NCDs represents a type of "global health whack-a-mole" problem, which now requires that at least equal global attention be paid to the NCDs.

I can still remember sitting in a small group meeting outside of Seattle a few years ago with Bill Gates and many of the leading thinkers involved with the GBD and related studies and hearing that one day the most cost-effective interventions to improve global health might be those directed against NCDs, possibly including increased tobacco taxation. Thus, the next "big picture" global health interventions may include constraining access to tobacco through public policies; mass treatment with "poly-pills" that would contain a statin component (to reduce blood cholesterol), an antihypertensive (to lower blood pressure), and aspirin (to anticoagulate blood); and environmental cleanup to reduce air pollution hazards. Indeed, a recent *Lancet* Commission predicting what the future of global health will look like in 2035 stresses the importance of using and expanding fiscal policies as "powerful and underused levers" to curb NCDs (as well as injuries) [11].

Sunset of the Millennium Development Goals (MDGs)

The MDGs ended in 2015, and in their place are soon to be launched a new set of 17 Sustainable Development Goals (SDGs). It is clear that great gains were made in the fight against childhood vaccine-preventable diseases and against AIDS and malaria as a result of massive deployment of lifesaving interventions, including vaccines, antiretroviral therapies, bed nets, and antimalarial drugs. As we will see in the next chapter, successes in the struggle against NTDs have been more modest. A key message that must be heard by global policymakers is the importance of not lapsing into complacency. These gains were hard-won and expensive. I am now concerned that when good health becomes merely 1 among 16 other SDGs, the emphasis that has been placed on health over the past 15 years will be diluted and will not continue in the coming decades.

Moreover, the apparent shift away from infectious and communicable diseases to the NCDs has created a new set of worries, as we face a rising tide of cancer, cardiovascular disease, chronic respiratory disease, diabetes, unipolar depression, and Alzheimer's disease. While this shift has been ascribed mostly to lifestyle changes, including tobacco use, I also believe there is a neglected component in the reported incidence of NCDs—one that is unique to poor countries. Specifically, many of the neglected tropical diseases are chronic, debilitating conditions that resemble NCDs, so some of the burden now being ascribed to NCDs may in fact be due to NTDs [12].

Some of the disease burden currently ascribed to NCDs among the poor may actually be caused by NTDs.

Therefore, we cannot tackle the NCDs without simultaneously taking on the NTDs. The exact burden of NCDs that can actually be ascribed to NTDs remains unmeasured, but it appears to be substantial given the fact that NTDs represent the most common afflictions of the poor. The importance of the NTDs and their special features that resemble NCDs will be discussed next. From there, we will see how these findings exposed a surprise burden of disease among the poor in wealthy countries.

Summary Points

1. Blue marble health refers to a shifting paradigm in global health in which the poor living in the world's wealthy countries account for most of the world's neglected diseases, including the NTDs, HIV/AIDS, tuberculosis, and malaria, as well as some important NCDs.

2. This paradigm shift follows from major changes in the global health landscape that began in 2000 following the launch of the United Nations Millennium Development Goals (MDGs), and with it, tens of billions of dollars in overseas development assistance for health in poor countries.

3. New measurements from the Global Burden of Disease Study have demonstrated powerful advances in global health, especially for MDGs 4 and 6.

4. Through MDG 4 and the creation of Gavi, vaccination coverage was extended widely in less developed countries, leading to substantial reductions in childhood deaths from measles, tetanus, diphtheria, whooping cough, Hib meningitis, and pneumococcal disease.

5. Similarly, through MDG 6, deaths from HIV/AIDS and malaria have decreased substantially as a result of large-scale programs, including PEPFAR, PMI, and GFATM.

6. Low-income countries, including those in sub-Saharan Africa, especially benefited from many of these MDG 4 and 6 interventions, possibly with some of the greatest gains seen in lowered mortality for certain childhood-preventable diseases, malaria, and HIV/AIDS occurring on the African continent.

7. However, the progress made against communicable and infectious diseases in the world's poorest countries exposed some unexpected global health shifts.

   a. First were the commensurate increases in NCDs, although some of that NCD burden may actually result from NTDs.

   b. Second was the surprising finding of widespread neglected diseases among the poor living in wealthy countries—the essential tenet of blue marble health.

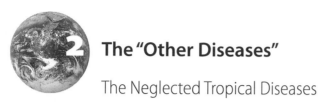

2 The "Other Diseases"

The Neglected Tropical Diseases

Through more than $70 billion in overseas development assistance from the G8 countries, together with international cooperation implemented within the framework of the UN Millennial Development Goals, dramatic reductions have been achieved in child mortality (MDG 4), and in deaths from HIV/AIDS and malaria (MDG 6). Progress toward MDG 4 was achieved first and foremost through increased vaccine coverage and global access to new vaccines for pneumococcus and rotavirus, while MDG 6 gains occurred mostly through increased access to essential medicines (antiretroviral drugs and antimalarial drugs) and bed nets. As a consequence of these great reductions in the deaths and DALYs from communicable and infectious diseases, particularly in Africa, the Global Burden of Disease Study 2010 determined that for the first time ever the global disease burden of noncommunicable diseases (NCDs), especially cancer, cardiovascular diseases, chronic pulmonary diseases, diabetes, unipolar depression, and Alzheimer's disease, now exceeds infectious diseases and represents the world's major causes of illness.

In light of these findings, the global health community was quick to place new emphasis on the control of NCDs as the next "big wave." Efforts to combat NCDs became especially urgent in the "Global South," meaning Africa, Asia, and Latin America. In response, the UN General Assembly organized a high-level meeting in New York to review and assess a 2011 political declaration on the NCDs [1]. In parallel, a *Lancet* Commission on investing in health (led by former World Bank chief economist, United States secretary of the treasury, and Harvard president Larry Summers together with University of Washington professor Dean Jamison) was also established to formulate plans for the next 20 years. The *Lancet* Commission found that fiscal policies directed at taxation of tobacco, alcohol, and other harmful substances, as well as those focused on reducing subsidies for fossil fuels linked to air pollution, might one day represent some of the most powerful pro–public health forces [2].

However, I believe that the apparent rise of the NCDs at the expense of declining infectious diseases partly ignores a harsh reality presented by the third (and often forgotten) component of MDG 6, which unfortunately was named "other diseases." In my previous book, *Forgotten People, Forgotten Diseases* [3], I explained how a group of these other diseases that I helped co-brand as the NTDs [4] actually represents the most common afflictions of the world's poor. Our original list of 13–14 major NTDs [5–7] was subsequently modified by the World Health Organization (WHO) to a list of 17 NTDs. However, our open access journal *Public Library of Science Neglected Tropical Diseases* (*PLOS NTDs*) has also shaped an expanded list that includes dozens more disease conditions.

NTDs are the most common diseases of the poor. Virtually every person on the planet living in extreme poverty is affected by at least one NTD.

The GBD 2013 has recently derived new estimates for the number of people actually infected with the 17 NTDs (as currently defined by WHO), and these are shown in table 2.1 [8]. In aggregate, there are more than two billion cases of NTDs worldwide, representing the most common diseases of people living in poverty. The major features of each of the leading NTDs (listed in order of prevalence) can be described as follows:

- *Ascariasis* is the most common NTD and possibly the most common affliction of the poor. Transmitted by the ingestion of parasite eggs that are nearly ubiquitous in the dirt found in impoverished rural and urban areas, ascariasis is caused by the roundworm *Ascaris lumbricoides,* which lives in the small intestines of millions of children. Chronic infection with *A. lumbricoides* produces malnutrition, which in turn leads to physical and cognitive growth delays. The larval stages of *A. lumbricoides* also migrate through the lungs to cause wheezing and a clinical syndrome that resembles asthma. The parasite is highly sensitive to deworming medication—typically mebendazole or albendazole—but because

Table 2.1 GBD 2013 estimates of the 17 diseases considered by WHO as NTDs

Rank	Disease	Prevalent cases in 2013 (in millions)	Common name	Major clinical features
1	Ascariasis[a]	804.4	Intestinal roundworm	Malnutrition (soil transmitted)
2	Trichuriasis[a]	477.4	Whipworm	Colitis (soil transmitted)
3	Hookworm disease[a]	471.8	Hookworm infection	Anemia (soil transmitted)
4	Schistosomiasis	290.6	Snail fever	Chronic liver and renal disease; female genital schistosomiasis; cancer (water-borne, snail transmitted)
5	Foodborne trematodiases	80.2	Liver fluke Lung fluke	Bile duct fibrosis, cancer Hemoptysis (coughing blood) (water-borne, snail transmitted)
6	Dengue	58.4[b]	Breakbone fever	Fever, shock, hemorrhage (mosquito transmitted)
7	Lymphatic filariasis	43.8	Elephantiasis	Limb and genital disfigurement (mosquito transmitted)
8	Onchocerciasis	17.0	River blindness	Blindness, skin disease (blackfly transmitted)
9	Chagas disease	9.4	Chagas disease	Cardiac enlargement, arrhythmias, aneurysms (kissing bug transmitted)
10	Leishmaniasis	4.0[c]	Kala-azar Aleppo evil	Leukemia-like illness Skin ulcer (sandfly transmitted)
11	Trachoma	2.4	Trachoma	Blindness
12	Cysticercosis	1.0	Cysticercosis	Epilepsy
13	Cystic echinococcosis	0.8	Hydatid cyst	Space-occupying lesions, liver, lung, kidneys
14	Leprosy	0.65	Leprosy	Skin and limb disfigurement
15	Rabies	0.06[d]	Rabies	Hydrophobia, coma, death
16	African trypanosomiasis	0.02	Sleeping sickness	Coma, death (tsetse transmitted)
17	Dracunculiasis	<0.01	Guinea worm	Lower limb disfigurement
18	Yaws	Not determined	Yaws	Skin and limb disfigurement
19	Buruli ulcer	Not determined	Buruli ulcer	Skin and limb disfigurement
	Total	2,260		

Source: Revised from data in [8], http://dx.doi.org/10.1016/S0140–6736(15)60692–4.
[a] WHO lists ascariasis, trichuriasis, and hookworm disease under the category of soil-transmitted (intestinal) helminth infections.
[b] Incident cases rather than prevalent cases.
[c] Both cutaneous and visceral forms.
[d] Incident cases not determined by GBD 2013 but estimates from [9].

the eggs are pervasive in the soil, the infection can return within a few months.

- *Trichuriasis* is a parasitic worm that lives for years in the colon, where it causes inflammation leading to colitis and dysentery in children with severe infections. The parasite eggs are also found in dirt. I have argued that the cause of trichuriasis, *Trichuris trichiura*, is the world's leading cause of inflammatory bowel disease. The treatment is the same as for ascariasis, but the medicines do not work as well, explaining why mass drug administration (MDA) is not as effective as it is for ascariasis. Reinfection also occurs.

- *Hookworm infection* or disease is mostly caused by *Necator americanus*, a small parasitic worm that lives for many years in the small intestines, where it extracts blood and causes intestinal blood loss. By this mechanism, hookworm infection is considered a major and global cause of iron deficiency anemia. Today, iron deficiency anemia is also an important cause of mortality as well as malnutrition, especially for children and women of reproductive age—two populations with low underlying iron reserves. In children, hookworm disease causes growth failure and intellectual and cognitive deficits, as well as loss in future wage earnings. Hookworm infection is also arguably the most common complication of pregnancy for women living in poverty. Pregnant women with hookworm experience high maternal morbidity and mortality, and their infants are at greater risk of adverse events, including death. MDA with albendazole and mebendazole is also not as effective as it is for ascariasis, and consequently I am leading an effort based at our Sabin Vaccine Institute and Texas Children's Hospital Center for Vaccine Development (and now expanded through a new European Union–based consortium known as HOOKVAC) to develop a human hookworm vaccine that is now in clinical trials in Brazil and Gabon.

- *Schistosomiasis* is a blood fluke infection resulting from *Schistosoma haematobium*, the cause of urogenital schistosomiasis, or *S. mansoni*, the cause of intestinal and hepatic schistosomiasis, as well as an Asian schistosome—*S. japonicum*. Snails are intermediate hosts of schistosomes, and infections are acquired through water contact where these carriers live. *S. haematobium* is now recognized as a major cause of urinary tract pathology and even bladder cancer (the parasite eggs are themselves carcinogens), in addition to chronic kidney disease. *S. haematobium* also causes female genital schistosomiasis, which I believe could be the most common gynecologic condition of women who live in poverty in Africa, as well as a major cofactor in Africa's AIDS epidemic. *S. mansoni* is a significant cause of chronic intestinal and liver dysfunction. MDA with a drug known as praziquantel is the major approach to controlling schistosomiasis in poor countries. The London-based Schistosomiasis Control Initiative is leading some of these efforts. However, MDA with praziquantel does not stop rein-fection. For that reason, at the Sabin Vaccine Institute we are also developing a schistosomiasis vaccine that is now in clinical trials. In addition, Brazil's Oswaldo Cruz Foundation and France's Institut Pasteur (Lille) and INSERM also have vaccines in clinical trials.

- *Foodborne trematodiases* are additional fluke infections transmitted by snails, but these are acquired by ingesting different intermediate hosts found in water, such as uncooked fish or crabs. Three species of liver fluke—*Clonorchis sinensis*, *Opisthorchis viverrini*, and *O. felineus*—are also carcinogens and represent major causes of bile duct carcinoma (also known as cholangiocarcinoma). Praziquantel, the drug used for schistosomiasis MDA, is also effective for most foodborne trematode infections.

- *Dengue* or dengue fever is a virus infection transmitted by *Aedes* mosquitoes found in urban settings in the tropics and subtropics. It is one of several so-called arboviral infections. Although listed among the NTDs, it does not typically produce chronic sequelae as do the other NTDs; moreover, dengue does not always dispropor-tionately affect the poor. I believe we are in the middle of a global dengue pandemic, with an explosion of new cases in Asia and the Americas, as well as Africa. Because there is a potential commercial market for dengue interventions, the major pharmaceutical compa-nies are leading international efforts to develop new dengue vaccines.

- *Lymphatic filariasis* (LF) is a parasitic worm infection (mainly *Wuchereria bancrofti*) transmitted by mosquitoes that can produce chronic and disfiguring lymphedema and hydrocele of the limbs, breasts, and genitals. The end-stage condition of LF, also known as elephantiasis, mainly affects adults, rendering them too sick for work. LF is also highly stigmatizing, especially for girls and women. The good news is that MDA through WHO's Global Programme to Eliminate LF, using either diethylcarbamazine citrate or ivermectin, together with albendazole, is actually interrupting transmission of LF, so the prevalence of this ancient NTD is now decreasing. It is forecast that LF could be eliminated by 2020.

- *Onchocerciasis,* also known as river blindness, is another parasitic worm infection, caused by *Onchercerca volvulus*. The disease is transmitted by blackflies that live near fast-flowing streams in impoverished areas, where it represents an important cause of blindness, but it is also a highly debilitating and disfiguring skin disease. Recently onchocerciasis has also been postulated to possibly cause epilepsy and a neurological condition of children known as "nodding syndrome." MDA with the drug ivermectin has made a big impact on reducing the prevalence and incidence of onchocerciasis, leading to elimination of the disease in the Americas (through the efforts of the Onchocerciasis Elimination Program for the Americas), while reducing its prevalence in Africa (through the African Programme for Onchocerciasis Control). In addition, the Sabin Vaccine Institute is sponsoring the Onchocerciasis Vaccine for Africa initiative, led by scientists in the United States, Europe, and Africa.

- *Chagas disease* is caused by a parasitic single-celled protozoan known as a trypanosome (*Trypanosoma cruzi*) that can invade the heart and cause debilitating heart disease. Also known as American trypanosomaisis, this disease is transmitted by triatomine "kissing bug" insects, but it is also passed on from mother to child. Chagas disease is considered a major cause of heart disease in Latin America, and recently scientists at the National School of Tropical Medicine at Baylor College of Medicine have found widespread transmission of the disease in Texas. The two major medicines used to treat Chagas disease—benznidazole and nifurtimox—are seldom used, because most Chagas patients live in extreme poverty and are not diagnosed. Even when patients do receive treatment for Chagas disease, however, the medicines can be quite toxic. Because long courses of therapy are required, often patients cannot tolerate a complete treatment course. The product development partnership

(PDP) Drugs for Neglected Diseases Initiative is pioneering the development and testing of new, more effective, and safer drugs for Chagas disease, while the Sabin Vaccine Institute and Texas Children's Hospital Center for Vaccine Development is developing a therapeutic vaccine that could be used alongside treatment. A Global Chagas Disease Coalition based in the Americas and Europe is leading advocacy and awareness efforts for this disease.

- *Leishmaniasis* is also caused by parasitic single-celled protozoa. More than a dozen different species of *Leishmania* parasites cause different syndromes of leishmaniasis. Visceral leishmaniasis, also known as kala-azar, is found mostly in India and East Africa and results in a severe leukemia-like illness that is highly fatal. Cutaneous leishmaniasis causes a disfiguring skin ulcer that affects populations in the Middle East, North Africa, Latin America, and elsewhere. Treatment of kala-azar using a medicine first developed to treat systemic fungal infections—liposomal amphotericin B—is expensive and not widely available. Treatment of cutaneous leishmaniasis can also be cumbersome and provides mixed results in terms of efficacy. Two PDPs—the Seattle-based Infectious Disease Research Institute and the Sabin Vaccine Institute and Texas Children's Hospital Center for Vaccine Development—are developing leishmaniasis vaccines.
- *Trachoma* is an important cause of blindness in impoverished areas, caused by an intracellular bacteria, *Chlamydia trachomitis*. Through the International Trachoma Initiative, based in Atlanta at the Task Force for Global Health, MDA with the antibiotic azithromycin is leading to dramatic reductions in prevalence that might one day lead to trachoma elimination, with an accelerated elimination timeline of 2020.

It should also be pointed out that many of the world's poor are simultaneously infected with multiple NTDs, especially ascariasis, trichuriasis, and hookworm infection, which are commonly known either as intestinal helminth infections (worms) or soil-transmitted helminth infections. Moreover, it is common for an individual with schistosomiasis, LF, or onchocerciasis to also have intestinal helminth infections. In short, the "bottom billion," are more often than not polyparasitized with multiple NTD pathogens.

NTDs Resemble NCDs

Together with Professor Abdallah Daar at the University of Toronto, we noted that many of the NTDs more closely resemble NCDs than they do typical infectious diseases that many Westerners experience [10]. This observation reflects the fact that most people who have contracted NTDs do not have access to treatment (or treatments have not yet been developed), and they therefore live with these illnesses for years, decades, or even their entire lives. Thus, many of the NTDs are long-standing and debilitating parasitic infections that over time produce significant end-organ damage. For example, as highlighted above, schistosomiasis can produce cirrhosis of the liver or chronic renal disease leading to kidney failure; Chagas disease can produce incapacitating heart disease and failure; hookworm infection can lead to moderate and severe anemia; onchocerciasis and trachoma can result in blindness; and LF, onchocerciasis, and Buruli ulcer can produce disfiguring skin disease. Moreover, some forms of both schistosomiasis and foodborne trematodiases are significant causes of cancer in some developing countries because the parasites or their eggs are actually carcinogens. For these reasons, at least some proportion of the NCDs among the poor is actually a result of chronic infection from NTDs. This is an important observation, because it suggests that lifestyle changes and taxation or other fiscal policies targeting NCDs may not get to the neglected root causes of the poor's long-term morbidities. There is an equally important need to directly tackle the NTDs.

Some of the disease burden currently ascribed to NCDs among the poor may actually be caused by NTDs.

NTDs, Poverty, and Human Development

Still another key observation about the impact of NTDs is that long-standing and chronic infections cause disabilities that have consequences beyond the realm of public health. The NTDs have the interesting but disturbing ability to cause poverty because they render people too sick to go to work (as is the case with LF, onchocerciasis, foodborne trematodiases, Buruli ulcer, and hookworm infection); or, they cause persistent infections in children that result in diminished intellectual and cognitive development and physical growth (as is the case for hookworm infection and schistosomiasis), ultimately leading to reductions in future wage earning [11, 12]. Moreover, hookworm and schistosomiasis disproportionately affect women of reproductive age and pregnant women, causing increased maternal morbidity and mortality, as well as poor neonatal outcomes [13]. NTDs also impair mental health [14] and can be highly stigmatizing because they can disfigure, as is the case for Buruli ulcer, onchocerciasis, LF, and leprosy (fig. 2.1) [15]. It is important to remember that these diseases are not rare conditions; virtually every person in poverty is believed to have at least one NTD. The NTDs represent a major but hidden reason that the bottom billion cannot escape poverty.

In order to emphasize the effects of NTDs on human development, Dr. Jennifer Herricks, a postdoctoral fellow, and I derived a "worm index" that uses numbers from WHO's Preventive Chemotherapy and Transmission Control database and combines national information for the number of children who require treatment for their intestinal helminth infections and schistosomiasis, together with the total population requiring treatment for LF [16]. As shown in figure 2.2, we found a strong and inverse association between a nation's worm index and its calculated human development index

Figure 2.1.
Public health banner to counter the stigma of
leprosy through awareness of treatment, at Brigade
Road construction site, Bangalore, India. From [15].

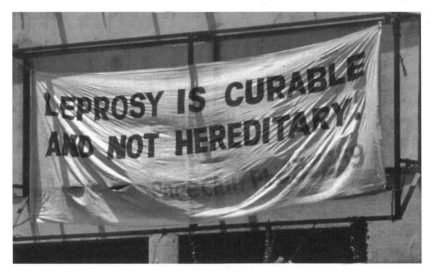

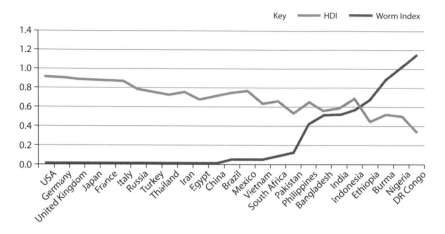

Figure 2.2.
Comparison of worm index versus the human
development index. From [16].

(HDI), a complex summary measure used by the United Nations Development Program that incorporates life expectancy, educational attainment,
and living standards.

One of the reasons for linking NTDs to human development is to ensure
that these diseases remain included within a new framework that follows on
the heels of the MDGs after 2015. The post-2015 MDGs "version 2.0" are
known as the Sustainable Development Goals (SDGs),
which came out of a UN conference on sustainable development held in Rio de Janeiro in 2012 (Rio+20) [17]. As
shown in figure 2.3, the SDGs have some overlap with
MDGs in terms of continuing global commitments to
poverty reduction (SDG 1), hunger (SDG 2), health (SDG
3), and empowering girls and women (SDG 5), but they
also place new emphases on the environment, including
climate change (SDG 13) and biodiversity (SDG 15), as well as water and
sanitation (SDG 6). A key priority for the NTD community of scientists and
public health officials is to keep these diseases on the radar screen of the
SDGs and to maintain the momentum that began in 2005 with efforts to
scale-up mass treatment for these conditions.

> *NTD control and
> elimination
> represents a highly
> cost-effective means
> of meeting new SDG
> goals and targets.*

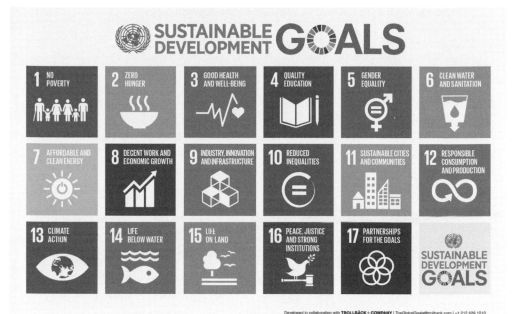

Figure 2.3. The United Nations' Sustainable Development Goals, 2016–2030. United Nations, http://www.un.org/sustainabledevelopment/sustainable -development-goals.

Mass Drug Administration and the London Declaration for NTDs

Since the late 1980s, efforts have been in place to provide mass treatment as a means to control or in some cases eliminate NTDs. The details of how mass drug administration is practiced is described in my previous book, *Forgotten People, Forgotten Diseases* [3]. Briefly, entire villages or districts in poor rural and some urban areas are provided pills that can either treat or prevent specific NTDs. The major NTDs targeted by MDA (now also known as "preventive chemotherapy" by WHO) are shown in table 2.2. A key point about the essential NTD medicines required to practice preventive chemotherapy is that most of them are donated by the major pharmaceutical companies, and in 2010 these companies reaffirmed their commitment to continue these donations for as long as necessary through a London Declaration for NTDs [18].

Table 2.2. Major NTDs targeted by MDA (preventive chemotherapy)

NTD	Treatment	Major donor pharmaceutical companies
Ascariasis, trichuriasis, hookworm infection	Albendazole mebendazole	GlaxoSmithKline Johnson & Johnson
Schistosomiasis	Praziquantel	Merck KgaA
Lymphatic filariasis	DEC Ivermectin	Eisai Merck & Co.
Onchocerciasis	Ivermectin	Merck & Co.
Trachoma	Azithromycin	Pfizer, Inc.

Because of the geographic overlap among these major NTDs and the fact that most impoverished populations are polyparasitized, in 2005, Professors David Molyneux at the Liverpool School of Tropical Medicine, Alan Fenwick at Imperial College London, and I proposed combining the medicines used for an MDA in a "rapid impact package," working through WHO in order to achieve specific disease control and elimination targets [5–7]. I believed it was possible that the donated package of medicines could be effective in interrupting transmission and eliminating some of the NTDs such as lymphatic filariasis (LF) and trachoma, and possibly onchocerciasis and ascariasis, although for certain intestinal helminth-related diseases, such as hookworm infection and trichuriasis, the package was only a temporary solution, because the drugs—albendazole and mebendazole—are not always highly effective against these two NTDs, especially when they are used in a single dose [19–22]. In addition, there is the problem of hookworm and schistosomiasis post-treatment reinfection within a few months [23]. However, the rapid impact package had enormous potential because of its effect on public health and its cost-effectiveness. Because the medicines were provided for free, the package could be administered for only 50 cents per person annually.

Throughout 2005, we worked with the US Congress and the George W. Bush administration so that by 2006 an NTD Program was initiated at the United States Agency for International Development (USAID). I believe that the results derived from this USAID program are every bit as effective as were the President's Emergency Plan for AIDS Relief and the Global Fund to Fight AIDS, Tuberculosis, and Malaria, but at far lower costs—now at about $100 million annually for the NTD Program versus approximately $8 billion annually for PEPFAR (fig. 2.4). In total, USAID has supported treatment for more than 450 million people in 32 countries, roughly equivalent to one billion NTD treatments over the past decade [24]. Because MDA can help interrupt the transmission of some NTDs, a key goal for the USAID NTD Program is to eliminate LF and trachoma by 2020. In parallel, the British Department for International Development (DFID) has sponsored the delivery of almost as many NTD treatments, together with private support from two nongovernmental organizations: the END Fund and Geneva Global. A Global Network for NTDs based at the Sabin Vaccine Institute has helped to lead advocacy and education efforts in the fight against these diseases.

MDA rapid-impact packages for NTDs have reached at least 450 million people in developing countries, which is now putting many countries on the path to the elimination of LF, onchocerciasis, and trachoma.

MDA programs are generally led by ministries of health in disease-endemic countries, mostly in Africa and Asia, together with implementation partners that include nongovernmental development organizations (such as the London-based Schistosomiasis Control Initiative at Imperial College and Helen Keller International) and USAID contractors (such as RTI International and FHI 360) and

Figure 2.4.
USAID Neglected Tropical Diseases Program funding allocations by fiscal year. http://www.neglected diseases.gov/funding/index.html.

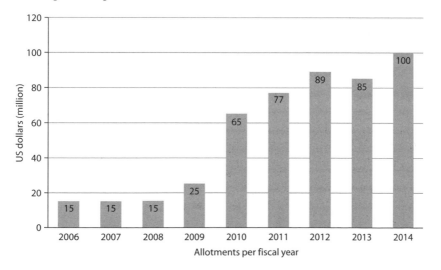

Table 2.3. Change in prevalence in NTDs targeted by rapid-impact package

Disease	% change from 1990 to 2013
Trachoma	−39.2
LF	−32.1
Onchocerciasis	−31.2
Ascariasis	−25.5
Trichuriasis	−11.6
Hookworm infection	−5.1
Schistosomiasis	+30.9

Source: [8], http://dx.doi.org/10.1016/S0140–6736(15)60692–4.

also with the guidance of WHO and its regional offices. An important point about these partnerships is that the ministries of health are themselves assuming leadership and in almost all cases providing an important level of financial support. However, the global community needs to do a better job of accurately determining the contributions made by the governments of the disease-endemic countries. For instance, for HIV/AIDS, substantial components of treatment activities and even funding come from the countries themselves.

MDA rapid-impact packages for NTDs are supporting the elimination of LF and trachoma, and are causing major reductions of onchocerciasis and ascariasis, but hookworm infection and schistosomiasis will require additional technological innovation, such as new anthelmintic vaccines.

In 2015, WHO published its finding that we are now reaching approximately 40% of people who require mass drug administration [25]. We have already helped 717 million people: this is an important achievement. But there is still work to do in order to treat an estimated 1.775 billion who require annual access to NTD medicines. In her important address to the 2015 World Health Assembly in Geneva, German Chancellor Angela Merkel highlighted the opportunity for combating the NTDs and bringing this problem to the agenda of the G7 nations. Accordingly, in 2015, I began spending time in Germany working with officials of the G7 in order to ensure that funds for drug programs that target the NTDs continue to be available.

Also in 2015, the GBD 2013 published estimates of the effectiveness of MDA and the treatment packages on reducing the prevalence of seven targeted NTDs [8]. It found that globally the prevalence of LF, trachoma, and onchocerciasis has been reduced by about 30–40%, while the

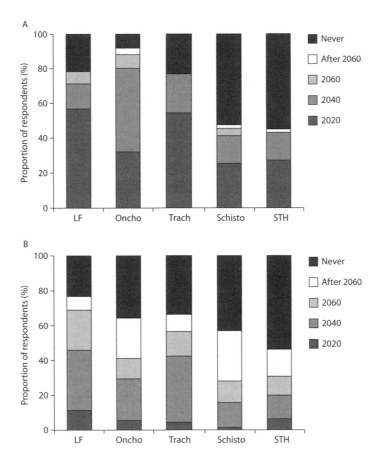

Figure 2.5.
Timeline for elimination (*top*) and eradication (*bottom*) for five
neglected tropical diseases—LF, onchocerciasis, trachoma,
schistosomiasis, and soil-transmitted helminth infections. From [26].

prevalence of ascariasis was reduced by 25%, confirming that we are on a good
path toward disease elimination. However, the global prevalence of hookworm infection has been reduced by only 5%, while the occurrence of schistosomiasis has actually increased by about 30% (table 2.3) [8]. The schistosomiasis numbers partly reflect the fact that only 13% of eligible populations are
currently receiving treatment. Accordingly, in 2013 we surveyed almost 400
experts, who concurred that the rapid impact package holds promise for eliminating LF, trachoma, and onchocerciasis, but not hookworm infection and
the other intestinal helminths or schistosomiasis (fig. 2.5) [26].

Next Steps

We are seeing fantastic reductions in the prevalence or incidence of LF, trachoma, onchoerciasis, and ascariasis, but less progress has been made against the other NTDs. For these reasons, we will need new technologies to combat hookworm infection (and possibly trichuriasis), schistosomiasis, and other NTDs. In the case of onchocerciasis, although reductions have been substantial, almost two decades of MDA will be required, so better technologies are also needed. Together with the leaders from nonprofit organizations committed to NTD research and development, including those from product development partnerships, we have highlighted the technologies that are most urgently needed [27]. As mentioned above, we are now developing a new generation of recombinant vaccines to prevent NTDs, including hookworm and schistosomiasis [28, 29]. These are biotechnologies that could be used alongside the rapid impact package. A recent study confirmed the cost-effectiveness of a hookworm vaccine used in conjunction with MDA [30].

Beyond the seven NTDs now being targeted by MDA, several other diseases that have enormous global health importance also exist: Dengue fever is a serious viral NTD transmitted by mosquitoes that has now reached the point of pandemic potential. Chagas disease is a debilitating cause of heart disease in the poor; it is a parasitic infection transmitted by kissing bugs. I will discuss both of these diseases in greater detail when addressing the NTDs in the Americas. Finally, leishmaniasis is a parasitic infection transmitted by sandflies, which is now affecting conflict zones in the Middle East and Africa. It will be further discussed as part of global vaccine diplomacy initiatives.

Summary Points

1. NTDs are the most common afflictions of people who live in extreme poverty, and all of the bottom billion are affected by at least one NTD.
2. These diseases are chronic and debilitating parasitic and related infections, which can resemble NCDs in terms of their effects on long-term end-organ damage.

3. The NTDs trap people in poverty because their debilitating effects lead to diminished worker productivity and negative pregnancy outcomes, as well as impaired child development.

4. NTDs are also inversely associated with human development, so NTD treatment and prevention efforts need to be incorporated in the new SDGs.

5. Seven of the most common NTDs are currently being targeted by MDA—ascariasis, trichuriasis, hookworm infection, schistosomiasis, LF, onchocerciasis, and trachoma—often in a rapid impact package of medicines that annually reaches hundreds of millions of people.

6. This approach is opening a path to the elimination of LF and trachoma, and in some cases onchocerciasis and ascariasis. For other NTDs, including hookworm infection, trichuriasis, and schistosomiasis, alternative or companion technologies will be required, such as anthelmintic vaccines. Improved technologies will also be needed for onchocerciasis in order to eliminate this disease over the next decade.

7. Together, USAID and DFID are supporting most of the costs of MDA treatment for the NTDs, but in 2015 German Chancellor Angela Merkel addressed the World Health Assembly in order to bring NTDs to the attention of the G7 countries.

Introducing Blue Marble Health

The framework of the NTDs first emerged following the launch of the UN's Millennial Development Goals. In 2005, tackling the NTDs was very much framed as a pro-poor strategy that targeted sub-Saharan Africa, and our original list of 13 diseases was based on the major NTDs affecting the African continent (box 3.1) [1]. But even then we recognized that NTDs were worldwide and important public health and economic problems of South and Southeast Asia, as well as the poorest countries of the Americas, including Bolivia, Guyana, Haiti, and in Central America, Guatemala, Honduras, and Nicaragua.

After first moving to Texas in 2011, I began to think about NTDs differently. Although we called them neglected *tropical* diseases, I found that the tropical component might be less important than the social determinants that give rise to these conditions. Instead, I came to realize that poverty was the overriding determinant engendering the NTDs. These diseases were found only in the setting of extreme poverty, but they also reinforce poverty through specific mechanisms: the NTDs interfere with worker productivity, child development, and women's health; they also can be highly stigmatizing.

The link between disease and a social determinant such as poverty had been highlighted before by Jeffrey Sachs, as well as by Dean Jamison and his colleagues in their landmark 1993 World Bank document—the *World Development Report*—that linked investments in health to economic returns on investment [2], and by the writings of Sir Michael Marmot in London on social determinants of health inequalities [3].

Box 3.1.

The Original List of 13 Neglected Tropical Diseases in Africa and Their Major Etiologic Agents

Protozoan Infections

African trypanosomiasis	*Trypanosoma gambiense,* *T. rhodesiense*
Kala-azar (visceral leishmaniasis)	*Leishmania donovani*

Helminth Infections

STH Infections

Ascariasis	*Ascaris lumbricoides*
Trichuriasis	*Trichuris trichiura*
Hookworm infection	*Necator americanus*

Schistosomiasis

Urinary schistosomiasis	*Schistosoma haematobium*
Hepatobiliary schistosomiasis	*S. mansoni*
Lymphatic filariasis	*Wuchereria bancrofti*
Onchocerciasis	*Onchocerca volvulus*
Dracunculiasis	*Dracunculus medinensis*

Bacterial Infections

Trachoma	*Chlamydia trachomitis*
Leprosy	*Mycobacterium leprae*
Buruli ulcer	*Mycobacterium ulcerans*

Driving through the poorest parts of Houston and elsewhere in Texas was a stark wake-up call that poverty was not unique to sub-Saharan Africa, or Asia, or even just the most destitute countries in Central and South America. Extreme poverty can be found even among the wealthiest economies, but the character of poverty in wealthy countries is unique. Unlike the poorest countries of Africa, or in Haiti, where poverty is almost universal, in wealthy countries poverty concentrates intensely in large pockets.

The way I began to look at poverty amidst wealth as it pertained to NTDs was to focus first on the Group of 20 (G20) economies. The G20 includes the European Union and 19 of the largest economies, led by the United States and followed by China, Japan, and Germany. The G20 was organized in 1999 in order to facilitate cooperation and communication following the Asian financial crisis, with its first summit held in 2008 during the global financial

Table 3.1. Updated economic indicators for the G20 nations and Nigeria

Country	GDP rank	2014 GDP (in trillions of US$)	Population rank
European Union	1	18.46	Not determined
United States	2	17.42	3
China	3	10.36	1
Japan	4	4.60	10
Germany	5	3.85	16
United Kingdom	6	2.94	22
France	7	2.83	21
Brazil	8	2.35	5
Italy	9	2.14	23
India	10	2.07	2
Russia	11	1.86	9
Canada	12	1.79	37
Australia	13	1.45	51
South Korea	15	1.41	27
Mexico	16	1.28	11
Indonesia	17	0.89	4
Turkey	19	0.80	18
Saudi Arabia	20	0.75	44
Nigeria	23	0.57	7
Argentina	25	0.54	32
South Africa	34	0.35	25
All G20 countries + Nigeria		66.95[a]	
Global		77.89	
% in G20 + Nigeria		86%	

Source: [5], doi:10.1371/journal.pntd.0003672.t001.
[a] Value obtained by adding the 2014 GDP dollars per country, then subtracting Germany, France, United Kingdom, and Italy, in order to avoid counting the numbers in the European Union twice.

crisis in that year [4]. I am captivated by the G20 because it boasts such enormous fiscal horsepower, with the capacity to introduce trillions of dollars in economic stimulus packages [4]. No other organization rivals it in terms of its ability to effect global change.

Shown in table 3.1 is a summary of the most recent economic indicators for the G20 countries, to which I have added the nation of Nigeria [5–8].

My rationale for adding Nigeria was to provide greater representation for sub-Saharan Africa beyond South Africa and the fact that the Nigerian economy, with a GDP of $570 billion, is far larger than that of South Africa. Overall, economists have determined that the world's gross domestic product (GDP), defined by the Organisation for Economic Co-operation and Development as "the standard measure of the value of final goods and services produced by a country during a period minus the value of imports" [9], was equivalent to US$77.9 trillion in the year 2014 [5–7]. Together, the G20 countries account for 86% of that global GDP [5].

Together, the G20 countries and Nigeria account for 86% of the global economy.

What strikes me the most about some of the countries with the largest GDPs—including Brazil, Mexico, China, and Saudi Arabia, where I have traveled and worked as part of my efforts to develop NTD vaccines—is how these nations are members of the G20 and have great wealth, yet simultaneously they host high levels of poverty. From firsthand experience, I recognized that these same nations also harbor widespread NTDs. For example, Brazil has the highest concentration of hookworm infection and schistosomiasis in the Americas; Mexico has the world's highest rates of mother-to-child Chagas disease transmission, while Argentina has the largest number of Chagas disease cases; China has one of the world's highest prevalences of ascariasis and foodborne trematodiases; and Saudi Arabia has endemic leishmaniasis.

Neither poverty nor NTDs are evenly distributed in the countries I just highlighted, nor are they evenly distributed in most of the G20 nations. Instead, poverty concentrates in specific areas of each G20 country. Shown in figure 3.1 is a map that highlights the concentrated pockets of poverty amidst the G20 economies, together with Nigeria [10, 11].

Poverty in the G20 nations is concentrated in specific areas of each of the blue marble countries.

In the following chapters, I will highlight the specific nature of poverty and the corresponding NTDs in each of the G20 countries and Nigeria—the major blue marble health nations. Briefly, among the Western Hemispheric G20 nations, poverty and disease concentrate in northern Argentina, northeastern Brazil and the Amazon region, southern Mexico, and the southern United States—especially in Texas and the Gulf Coast. In Asia and Oceania, the major impoverished areas in the G20 include western and southern

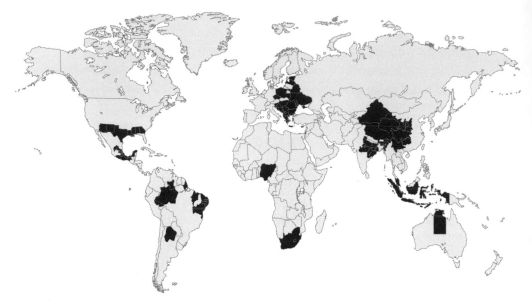

Figure 3.1.
Map of blue marble health shows areas of extreme poverty
concentrated amidst wealth in the G20 countries and Nigeria.
From [11]; map prepared by Esther Inman.

China, northern India, Indonesia, and the Northern Territory of Australia. Poverty is prevalent in eastern Europe, South Africa, and Nigeria [10, 11]. In contrast, certain G20 countries such as France, Germany, and the United Kingdom are not considered major sources of NTDs.

NTDs and Blue Marble Health

I first published the framework of blue marble health in an article titled "The Disease Next Door" in the international affairs journal *Foreign Policy* in March 2013 [10], and it was based on my findings that most of the world's NTDs paradoxically can be found in the G20 nations and Nigeria, predominantly in the concentrated areas mentioned above. The concept of blue marble health counters prevailing concepts of global health focused on the split between developed countries in the "Global North," that is, North America,

Europe, and Japan, and less developed countries in the "Global South," that is, Africa, Asia, and Central and South America. In its place, the poor living in specific areas of poverty in otherwise wealthy countries are accounting for the lion's share of neglected diseases.

As we will see, the world is changing in the sense that all economies are advancing and sustaining growth, even in Africa, but left behind is a bottom contingent that suffers daily from NTDs and related neglected infections. The blue marble invokes an iconic image of Earth taken by the crew of Apollo 17—Commander Eugene Cernan and pilots Ronald Evans and Harrison Schmitt—as they orbited the moon in December 1972, and which for a time was an international symbol for peace and healing (fig. 3.2) [11, 12].

Shown in table 3.2 is my initial analysis of the NTDs in the G20 nations and Nigeria, based on published data collected from papers written by academic authors and scientists, as well as from the Preventive Chemotherapy and Transmission (PCT) Control database from WHO, in addition to WHO leprosy data [10, 11]. The studies show that most of the world's visceral leishmaniasis cases—a serious, high-mortality protozoan parasitic NTD endemic to South Asia and eastern Africa (and some

Blue marble health represents a changing global health framework. It says that most of the world's NTDs and neglected diseases occur among the poor who live in wealthy countries, and this finding provides new opportunities for both poverty reduction and disease elimination.

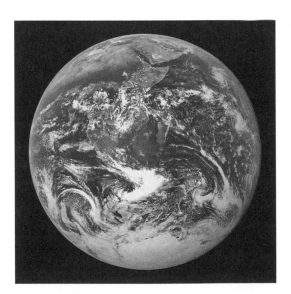

Figure 3.2.
The "blue marble"—an international symbol of peace and healing—as photographed by astronauts Eugene Cernan, Ronald Evans, and Jack Schmitt on December 7, 1972. From http://visibleearth.nasa.gov/view.php?id=55418; doi:10.1371/journal.pntd.0002570.g002.

Table 3.2. Selected NTDs in the G-20 countries and Nigeria

Country	GDP rank	Cases of visceral leishmaniasis reported	Cases of schistosomiasis	Cases of hookworm infection	Population requiring MDA for lymphatic filariasis	Cases of foodborne trematodiases	Registered cases of leprosy	Cases of Chagas disease
United States	1							0.3 million
China	2	378	0.8 million	39 million		38 million	2,468	
Japan	3					<1 million		
Germany	4							
France	5	18						
Brazil	6	3,481	1.5 million	32 million	2 million		29,690	1.9 million
United Kingdom	7							
Italy	8	134						
Russia	9					<1 million		
India	10	34,918		71 million	610 million		83,187	
Canada	11							<0.1 million
Australia	12						7	
Mexico	14	7		<1 million			480	1.1 million
South Korea	15					1–2 million	265	
Indonesia	16		<0.1 million	62 million	123 million		23,169	
Turkey	18	29						
Saudi Arabia	20	34	<0.1 million	<1 million			5	
Argentina	27	8		2 million			723	1.6 million
South Africa	29		4.9 million	5 million				
Nigeria	40	1	28.8 million	38 million	106 million			
Total cases in G20+Nigeria		39,008 reported	36 million	249 million	841 million	40 million	139,994	4.9 million
Total cases globally		58,227 reported	207 million	576 million	1.392 billion	56 million	181,941	8 million
% of cases in G20+Nigeria		67%	17%	43%	60%	71%	77%	61%

Source: [11], doi:10.1371/journal.pntd.0002570.t002.

parts of southern Europe, North Africa and the Middle East, and the Americas) exhibit the highest prevalence in G20 countries. Similarly, most of the world's Chagas disease cases—another parasitic protozoan NTD that causes debilitating heart disease—are in G20 countries, as are leprosy and most of the foodborne trematodiases—a common cause of cancer and other end-organ morbidities. Almost one-half of the hookworm cases are also found in G20 nations. These diseases represent the NTDs with the highest disease burden, as determined by the Global Burden of Disease Studies of 2010 and 2013, and they were selected on that basis [13, 14].

Shown in table 3.3 are updated numbers from the WHO PCT database obtained for the year 2013, which includes estimates of school-age children who require mass drug administration for their intestinal helminth infections and schistosomiasis, as well as total populations who require MDA for LF and onchocerciasis [5, 15–21]. It was found that one-half of these global helminth infections occurred among populations living in the G20 countries and Nigeria. These same helminth infections also account for almost 50% of the global disease burden of the NTDs [15], and these data were used to derive the worm index of human development [22] described in chapter 2. It was further found that the worm index is positive in six of the G20 countries—Brazil, China, India, Indonesia, Mexico, and South Africa—in addition to Nigeria [5].

Most of the world's NTDs with the highest disease burdens—including helminth infections, leishmaniasis, Chagas disease, leprosy, and dengue—are found predominantly in G20 countries and Nigeria.

As shown in table 3.4, outside of the helminth infections, updated numbers indicate that most of the world's cases of dengue fever now occur in the G20 countries and Nigeria [23]. By some accounts, we are in the midst of a dengue pandemic with more than 50 million incident cases in 2013 according to the GBD 2013 [14], but there may be as many as 390 million incident cases if so-called non-apparent cases are included [23]. Finally, updated WHO data also confirm that leprosy also predominates among the G20 and is still very much a blue marble health disease [24].

The finding that most of the world's highest-burden NTDs, including the major helminth infections linked to the worm index of human development, foodborne trematodiases leishmaniasis, Chagas disease, dengue, and leprosy, are found in the G20 wealthy economies and Nigeria has important implications for both public health and public policy. They include the

Table 3.3. Helminth infections among the G20 nations and Nigeria (2013)

Country	Total helminth infections
European Union	<0.1 million
United States	0
China	18.7 million
Japan	0
Germany	0
France	0
United Kingdom	0
Brazil	10.5 million
Italy	0
Russia	0
India	646.6 million
Canada	0
Australia	0
South Korea	0
Mexico	7.4 million
Indonesia	148.0 million
Turkey	0
Saudi Arabia	0
Argentina	0
Nigeria	234.0 million
South Africa	5.1 million
All G20 countries + Nigeria	1.0703 billion
Global	2.1349 billion
% in G20 + Nigeria	50%

Source: [5], doi:10.1371/journal.pntd.0003672.t002.
Note: Total helminth infections were calculated by adding the number of school-age children requiring treatment for soil-transmitted helminth infections and schistosomiasis, together with the total population requiring treatment for lymphatic filariasis and onchocerciasis. All of these numbers were based on the 2013 WHO PCT database, together with newly released information on onchocerciasis from WHO.

likelihood that the bottom economic tiers of societies are suffering from NTDs and as a result are remaining trapped in poverty. Because NTDs promote poverty, it is possible that one of the most efficient ways to raise

Table 3.4. Other high disease burden NTDs in the G20 countries

Country	Dengue in 2010	Leprosy (registered prevalence) in 2013
European Union	None reported	None reported
United States	None reported	289
China	6,523,946	1,908
Japan	None reported	2
Germany	None reported	None reported
France	None reported	None reported
United Kingdom	None reported	None reported
Brazil	5,371,268	28,485
Italy	None reported	None reported
Russia	None reported	None reported
India	32,541,392	86,147
Canada	None reported	None reported
Australia	None reported	0
South Korea	None reported	210
Mexico	1,987,320	451
Indonesia	7,590,213	19,730
Turkey	None reported	None reported
Saudi Arabia	152,009	4
Argentina	254,470	538
Nigeria	4,153,338	3,626
South Africa	None reported	None reported
All G20 countries + Nigeria	58,573,956	141,390
Global	96 million	180,618
% in G20 + Nigeria	61%	78%

Source: [5], doi:10.1371/journal.pntd.0003672.t003.

the economic level of each of the G20 countries would be to control and eliminate their NTDs internally. For me, the implications also include accountability and the opportunity for each of the leaders of the G20 nations

Blue marble health provides a new framework for shaping policy among the world's most powerful nations.

to take greater responsibility for their countries' own endemic and homegrown NTDs, with respect to disease control and elimination [5]. In so doing, at least one-half of the world's NTD disease burden could be dissolved. There is also an important research and development dimension for blue marble health, as many of the affected countries have a robust biotechnology infrastructure. These nations could recommit to developing new interventions that are required to combat their own NTDs, including new drugs, diagnostics, and vaccines [25, 26].

HIV/AIDS, TB, Malaria, and Blue Marble Health

Does the blue marble health concept extend beyond the NTDs? My analysis of 2014 data from WHO suggests that blue marble health is also highly relevant to "the big three" diseases: HIV/AIDS, TB, and malaria [27]. Shown in table 3.5 is my analysis and summary [27] of data from the year 2013 released in 2014 from WHO and United States Center for Disease Control and Prevention (CDC) [28–33].

Briefly, data from *The Gap Report* of UNAIDS and CDC indicate that 44% of the 35 million people living with HIV/AIDS live in G20 countries and Nigeria [27], although this figure is an underestimate because *The Gap Report* does not include data for China and Russia, both important countries in terms of HIV/AIDS [28, 29]. Similarly, 57% of the 11 million tuberculosis cases are living in G20 countries [27], but these

The G20 nations and Nigeria account for approximately one-half of the world's AIDS, TB, and malaria cases.

numbers also represent underestimates, as the *WHO Global Tuberculosis Report 2014* does not report specific data from Australia, Canada, Mexico, and South Korea [30, 31]. Finally, my analysis of the *WHO World Malaria Report 2014* finds that 45% of the world's malaria cases were also reported from G20 countries and Nigeria [27], although Nigeria and India accounted for the vast majority of these cases, in addition to 10 million cases each in China and Indonesia [32, 33]. The bottom line here is that the blue marble countries—the G20 and Nigeria—account for roughly one-half of the world's HIV/AIDS, tuberculosis, and malaria cases and at least one-half of the world's NTDs.

Table 3.5. HIV/AIDS, TB, and malaria among the G20 nations and Nigeria

Country	Economic rank	People living with HIV/AIDS in 2013	Tuberculosis prevalence in 2013	Suspected malaria cases in 2013
European Union (EU)	1	1,100,000	460,000	1,864,593
United States	2	1,200,000	10,000	1,500–2,000 annually
China	3	Not reported	1,300,000	5,555,001
Japan	4	Not reported	Not reported	None reported
Germany	5	See EU	See EU	See EU
France	6	See EU	See EU	See EU
United Kingdom	7	See EU	See EU	See EU
Brazil	8	730,000	110,000	1,893,018
Italy	9	See EU	See EU	See EU
Russia	10	Not reported	160,000	None reported
India	11	2,100,000	2,600,000	127,891,198
Canada	12	Not reported	Not reported	None reported
Australia	13	28,000	Not reported	None reported
South Korea	15	Not reported	Not reported	443
Mexico	16	180,000	Not reported	1,017,508
Indonesia	17	640,000	680,000	3,197,890
Turkey	19	See EU	See EU	255,125
Saudi Arabia	20	Not reported	Not reported	1,309,783
Argentina	22	Not reported	Not reported	4,913
Nigeria	25	3,200,000	570,000	21,659,831
South Africa	34	6,300,000	380,000	603,932
All G20 countries + Nigeria		15.5 million	6.3 million	165 million
Global		35 million	11 million	367 million
% in G20 + Nigeria		44%	57%	45%

Source: [29], http://dx.doi.org/10.1016/j.micinf.2015.05.004.

NCDs and Blue Marble Health

My final analysis, conducted in collaboration with Dr. Larry Peiperl at *PLOS Medicine*, indicates that in addition to all of the neglected diseases—NTDs plus HIV/AIDS, TB, and malaria—the concept of blue marble health ap-

Table 3.6. NCD mortality estimates in G20 countries + Nigeria, 2012

Country	GDP rank	Age-standardized death rate per 100,000 from NCDs in males	Age-standardized death rate per 100,000 from NCDs in females	Total deaths from NCDs in 2012 (in millions)
European Union	1			
United States	2	488.9	350.1	2.3
China	3	650.6	508.5	8.6
Japan	4	333.3	173.5	0.9
Germany	5	447.8	295.1	0.8
United Kingdom	6	425.9	302.2	0.5
France	7	412.7	234.8	0.5
Brazil	8	617.7	429.4	1.0
Italy	9	382.1	242.5	0.5
India	10	785.0	586.6	5.9
Russia	11	1,155.6	573.8	1.8
Canada	12	378.6	268.0	0.2
Australia	13	359.9	253.0	0.1
South Korea	15	415.0	221.4	0.2
Mexico	16	539.5	410.9	0.5
Indonesia	17	774.6	600.2	1.1
Turkey	19	726.3	430.8	0.4
Saudi Arabia	20	622.4	472.2	0.1
Nigeria	23	712.8	638.4	0.5
Argentina	25	599.4	370.9	0.3
South Africa	34	902.8	587.4	0.3
All G20 countries + Nigeria				26.5
Global				38
% of global NCD deaths occurring in the G20 + Nigeria				70%

Source: [36], doi:10.1371/journal.pmed.1001859.t001.

plies also to the noncommunicable diseases [34]. WHO's *Global Status Report on NCDs 2014* indicates that of the 56 million people who died in the year 2012, 38 million died from NCDs, with four major disease conditions—cancer, cardiovascular disease, chronic respiratory diseases, and diabetes—

accounting for more than 80% of those deaths [35]. About one-half of the deaths are from cardiovascular diseases, followed by cancer as the next leading cause [35]. As shown in table 3.6, the G20 countries and Nigeria also account for 70% of those NCD-related deaths, with the BRICS countries—Brazil, Russia, India, China, South Africa—responsible for roughly two-thirds of the G20/Nigeria deaths [34].

More than two-thirds of the major NCD deaths also occur in the G20 countries and Nigeria.

In *PLOS Medicine* we suggested that blue marble health could represent a convergence of three trends. Prior to the progress linked to the Millennium Development Goals, the neglected diseases—NTDs, HIV/AIDS, TB, and malaria—were thought of as the major purview of low-income countries in Africa and South Asia, but they are now widespread among the poor in G20 countries; whereas NCDs, conditions once considered diseases of the rich, are also now occurring among this same population. Since then, the world has changed, with all roads pointing to the poor living amidst wealth as the new global reservoir of poverty and disease (fig. 3.3). At least one study confirms that NCDs disproportionately occur among individuals with lower socioeconomic status, such that NCDs "are not necessarily diseases of the wealthy" [36].

A second level of convergence that needs to be considered is the co-endemicity of neglected diseases with NCDs. For example, it has been noted

Figure 3.3.
Blue marble health as a convergence of three trends.

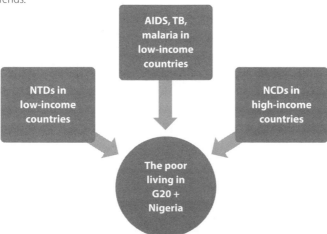

that diabetes and tuberculosis or diabetes and dengue comorbidities are common, especially among the poor [37, 38], but there are many other demonstrated and plausible associations and links. Increasingly, we can expect to see new syndromes arise as a consequence of neglected disease/NCD comorbid conditions.

Neglected disease/ NCD comorbid conditions may become the "new normal" among the poor living in the G20 and Nigeria.

In the following chapters we will look at blue marble health scenarios as they pertain to individual countries and regions and then identify common trends and themes that can be shaped into relevant public policy for the G20 nations and Nigeria.

Summary Points

1. The NTDs were originally conceived as African poverty-related diseases and subsequently incorporated diseases of the extreme poor in South and Southeast Asia and in Central and South America.
2. New evidence identifies a surprising burden of NTDs among the poor living in concentrated areas of poverty in wealthy G20 economies and Nigeria.
3. Most of the world's helminth infections, Chagas disease, leishmaniasis, dengue, and leprosy are found in G20 economies and Nigeria.
4. Approximately one-half of the world's "big three diseases" are also found in G20 economies in Africa.
5. Approximately 70% of NCDs are found in these same countries.
6. We may be seeing a convergence of three trends—NTDs, the big three diseases, and NCDs—are now occurring among the same population. All roads point to the poor living amidst wealth as the global reservoir of poverty and disease.
7. A second level of convergence that needs to be considered is the co-endemicity of neglected diseases with NCDs and new comorbid conditions.
8. One of the most efficient ways to raise the economic level of each of the G20 countries may be to control and eliminate their neglected infectious diseases and NCDs internally.
9. We need each of the G20 nations to take greater responsibility for its own indigenous (autochthonous) NTDs, with respect to disease

control and elimination. In so doing, at least one-half of the world's neglected disease burden could be dissolved.

10. There is also an important research and development implication for blue marble health, as many of the affected countries also have a robust biotechnology infrastructure. Blue marble health nations could recommit to developing new interventions that are required to combat their own NTDs, including new drugs, diagnostics, and vaccines.

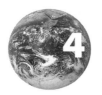

4 East Asia: China, Indonesia, Japan, and South Korea

There are five blue marble health countries in Asia, and all of them except India are found in East Asia. The story of East Asia's neglected diseases is a good representation of the tenets of blue marble health—namely, explosive economic growth in postwar Japan and Korea, as well as in eastern China following economic reforms that began during the 1980s, with each economic jump associated with dramatic reductions in the prevalence of NTDs and malaria. Nevertheless, significantly large areas have been left behind and are not benefiting from such successes, including southwestern China, Indonesia, and North Korea. These regions remain plagued by widespread NTDs.

China

The People's Republic of China is the world's second-largest and fastest-growing economy today. China's economic and market reforms began in the 1980s with the ascendancy and leadership of Deng Xiaoping. According to the World Bank, China's recent GDP economic growth has averaged 10% annually, and in so doing has lifted half a billion people out of poverty, while attaining most if not all its Millennium Development Goals [1]. Despite such gains, a crushing level of poverty persists. Data from 2011 show that 6.3% of China's population lives below the 2005–14 World Bank poverty level of $1.25 per day [2], while 18.6% live on less than $2 per day [3]. With a population greater than 1.3 billion, there are more than 200 million people who live on virtually nothing in China.

China's poverty is unevenly distributed. Not many of those 200 million destitute Chinese live in the amazing cities in the eastern part of the country with populations of more than five million people each—Beijing, Shanghai, Tianjin, Taipei, Nanjing, Wuhan, Shenyang, and Hangzhou; nor in a new megalopolis being created around Beijing and known as Jing-Jin-Ji, which comprises a population six times larger than the New York City metro area [4]; nor in the southeast in or near Guangdong Province (Pearl River Delta)—Dongguan, Guangzhou, Hong Kong, and Shenzhen. Instead, as shown in figure 4.1 [5], the economy of China exhibits a distinct east-to-west gradient of poverty.

Let's look at some of China's poorest provinces, particularly those in the southwest corner—Sichuan, Yunnan, Guizhou, Guangxi, and Hainan Provinces. Here, where many of China's "bottom 200 million" live, NTDs remain widespread, led by the intestinal helminth infections. Between 2001 and

Figure 4.1.
China's east-to-west poverty gradient.
From [5].

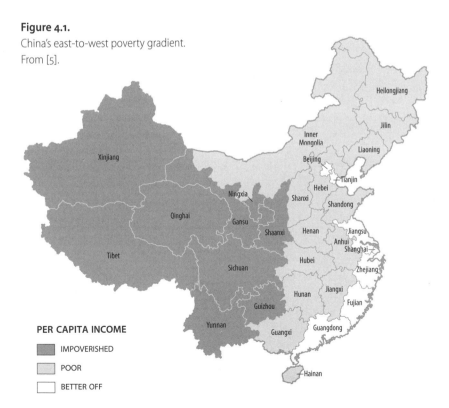

2004, the Chinese Center for Disease Control and Prevention, including its Institute of Parasitic Diseases based in Shanghai, conducted fecal examinations on more than 350,000 individuals in 687 study sites across China to reveal that almost 13% of its population (more than 150 million cases) is infected with *Ascaris* worms [6, 7]. However, like China's poverty, the distribution of ascariasis (as well as other intestinal helminth infections) in China is uneven. According to a study led by the Chinese CDC in collaboration with Swiss Tropical and Public Health Institute and the University of Basel, China's human ascariasis cases are concentrated in some of the same southwestern provinces where extreme poverty is still rampant, namely, Sichuan, Yunnan, and Guizhou Provinces, as well as in Hubei (north [*bei*] of the lake [*hu*]) and Hunan (south [*nan*] of the lake), two of the Yangtze River provinces where there is also a serious level of poverty [6, 7]. These studies were led in part by Xiao-Nong Zhou, who heads the Shanghai Institute, and Juerg Utzinger, who recently became director of the Swiss Institute.

The reason that poverty is such an important social determinant for intestinal helminth infections is still not entirely known. The life cycle of ascariasis is propagated when parasite eggs in the feces are shed in the environment. Included among the potential social and environmental determinants that arise from poverty are inadequate disposal of feces in poor areas, in some cases from open and indiscriminate defecation, as well as China's dependence on human feces as fertilizer, sometimes referred to as "night soil" [8]. Recently, in-depth and qualitative interviews were conducted in six rural villages in Guizhou, one of China's poorest provinces, in order to better understand the high intestinal helminth burden there [9]. Three major observations were made from that study, including (1) a low level of awareness about the existence of intestinal helminth infections among the villagers, (2) "local myths" about intestinal worms—that worms are essential for digestion and deworming drugs can cause infertility, and (3) overall low levels of village health care [9]. Furthermore, a recent extensive study conducted in Guizhou by researchers at the Chinese Academy of Sciences, the Chinese CDC, and Stanford University and published in *PLOS NTDs* reveals that intestinal helminth infections in children are strongly linked to poor cognition and school performance, as well as to childhood malnutrition [10].

Both extreme poverty and widespread NTDs are prevalent and reinforce each other in China's southwestern provinces.

What about some of China's other impoverished western provinces such as Xinjiang, Tibet, and Qinghai, where ascariasis rates are very low? In these areas there is low overall rainfall, with often dry or desertlike conditions that fail to promote the environmental stages of *Ascaris* infection required to continue the parasite life cycle. Thus, poverty is a critical factor, but not the only one, and climate still plays an important role in parasite transmission and disease ecology.

In regard to China's other major helminth infections that contribute to its worm index—schistosomiasis and LF—the nation has made impressive strides. China launched a national control program against schistosomiasis in the 1950s, with the result that today approximately only 300,000 cases remain (down from more than 10 million) along the Yangtze River and its tributaries and two drainage lakes, Poyang and Dongting [11, 12]. However, for those last remaining cases, elimination targets have been elusive, and new acute cases of the disease still reemerge among some local villages [11, 12]. Because Asian schistosomiasis (*Schistosoma japonicum* infection) is a zoonotic disease linked to water buffalo animal reservoirs, there is an effort to replace them with tractors and also to educate fishermen and others with extensive water contact not to defecate into bodies of water linked to the Yangtze River, where *Oncomelania* snail intermediate hosts still live [11]. There is optimism that schistosomiasis can eventually be wiped out, just as LF was previously eliminated (toward the end of the twentieth century), by MDA with diethylcarbamazine citrate. On the other hand, China still has more than 10 million cases each of two serious foodborne trematodiases (fluke infections), clonorchiasis and paragonimiasis [5, 12]. *Clonorchis* liver flukes are carcinogens that cause bile duct carcinoma, while *Paragonimus* lung flukes can cause severe tissue damage. Other serious zoonotic NTDs found in poor areas of China include both alveolar and cystic echinococcosis and cysticercosis [12].

In China, foodborne trematodiases are emerging as important causes of chronic diseases that resemble NCDs, even cancer.

Finally, vector-borne neglected diseases remain important in China. Rates of malaria have diminished considerably, partly with support from the Global Fund to Fight AIDS, Tuberculosis, and Malaria, to the point where this disease may soon be moving into its elimination phase in China [13]. However, there are concerns about the reintroduction of malaria in the island province of Hainan in the South China Sea, and malaria is still an important public health threat in Yunnan, on the border with Burma [14]. Serious arboviral infections found in China include Japanese encephalitis and dengue, with more focal distribution of tick-borne encephalitis in some of China's northern provinces near Mongolia, and Crimean-Congo hemorrhagic fever in the province of Xinjiang [15]. Similar to the intestinal helminth infections, Japanese encephalitis is believed to have shifted from an eastern coastal distribution to the central and western regions over the past fifty years, while dengue is distributed primarily in southern provinces [15]. Prominent among other viral infections in China is human rabies transmitted by dog bites—approximately 2,000 human rabies cases occur annually [16].

Noncommunicable diseases (NCDs) have become the most serious health threat to China, causing an estimated 8.6 million deaths annually [17]. However, the NTDs remain important poverty-promoting illnesses in China's southwest, and clonorchiasis is now a significant cause of cancer, thus underscoring the NTD and NCD link. The manner in which the patterns of NTDs and NCDs in China will evolve over the next few decades is of great interest. A 2010 Chinese census indicates that the nation faces a number of interesting demographic changes, marked by low fertility (and slower population growth) and a rapidly increasing elderly segment of the population, as well as accelerating urbanization [18]. Therefore, it can be expected that NCDs will remain China's predominant public health problem, but foodborne trematodiases and other NTDs will also remain. We also found that in some provinces, hookworm is a particularly important problem among the elderly, so this NTD may persist in the absence of new interventions [19].

Indonesia

Indonesia is a G20 emerging economy with a GDP approaching $1 trillion, the largest in Southeast Asia. At the same time, the World Bank classifies Indonesia as a lower-middle-income country, with almost one-half of the population living on less than $2 per day (and 18% on less than $1.25 per day) [20]. Thus, Indonesia's economic growth has left behind approximately 111 million people living in extreme poverty [21]. In a *PLOS NTDs* article we wrote in 2014, "Indonesia: An Emerging Market Economy Beset by Neglected

Table 4.1. The major neglected tropical diseases of Indonesia

Disease	Number of cases or people at risk	% of global disease burden or population at risk	Comments
Trichuriasis	95 million	16	STH infections in 31 of 33 provinces in Indonesia
Ascariasis	90 million	11	STH infections in 31 of 33 provinces in Indonesia
Hookworm infection	62 million	11	STH infections in 31 of 33 provinces in Indonesia
Schistosomiasis	25,000–50,000 at risk	<1	All cases in Central Sulawesi Province
Lymphatic filariasis	125 million at risk	9	Highest prevalence in eastern Indonesia
Leprosy	20,023 new cases in 2011	9 (of new global cases in 2011)	Especially in Central and West Java
Yaws	8,039 cases reported in 2009	Not determined	Highly endemic in Papua, Southeast Sulawesi, and Nusa Tenggara Timur provinces
Leptospirosis	Not determined	Not determined	
Dengue	3,436 deaths	58 (of the deaths in Southeast Asia); 23 (of deaths globally)	Indonesia has the second-largest number of cases worldwide
Chikungunya and Japanese encephalitis	Not determined	Not determined	

Source: [21], doi:10.1371/journal.pntd.0002449.t001.

Tropical Diseases (NTDs)," we indicated that most of that "bottom 111 million" is infected with at least one NTD [21].

Shown in table 4.1 is a listing of those NTDs, with the approximate numbers of cases taken from that paper [21]. Practically every person living in extreme poverty is infected with intestinal helminths or living in an area endemic for LF, or both. Updated information from the WHO PCT database indicates that almost 50 million school-age children in Indonesia require MDA for their intestinal helminth infections [22], while 100 million people need treatment for LF [23], with the result that Indonesia requires frequent rounds of MDA [24]. Today, Indonesia has an extremely high worm index, one of the highest in Asia.

Another unusual feature of LF in Indonesia is that it is the only country to host all three helminthic parasite species known to cause the disease—*Wuchereria bancrofti, Brugia malayi,* and *B. timori* [21]. Accordingly, MDA efforts will need to expand considerably if Indonesia hopes to eliminate LF and reduce the prevalence of its intestinal helminth infections. Only about one-half of the eligible population in the major endemic districts of Indonesia is treated regularly for LF [23], partly as a result of the incredibly complicated logistics required to reach remote regions in the country's 17,000 islands, along with compliance issues that partly stem from the social stigma linked to LF [21].

Indonesia's vast island geography is an impediment to MDA for its NTDs. This problem is compounded by inadequate budget allocations and decentralization.

However, a second major reason has been inconsistent governmental budget allocations as a result of inefficiencies associated with decentralization or lack of political will [21]. Yet even under these circumstances, a proof of concept has been achieved for the local elimination of LF in a region of eastern Indonesia [24]. The Indonesian Ministry of Health could improve in the intestinal helminth department—fewer than 10% of Indonesia's children who need MDA actually receive it on a periodic and frequent basis [22]. Moreover, Asian schistosomiasis (*S. japonicum* infection) is still also found focally in the Central Sulawesi part of the country.

Two important bacterial NTDs are still widespread among the poor in Indonesia: yaws and leprosy. Both of these diseases can produce highly disfiguring and stigmatizing conditions. Yaws is endemic in at least five Indonesian provinces, although efforts have begun to apply MDA through use of azithromycin, the same antibiotic used for MDA efforts against trachoma. Leprosy is still found in Java, and it is cause for concern that Indonesia still accounts for 10% of the world's new cases of the disease [21].

Of even greater concern is widespread dengue fever. Today, Indonesia accounts for a substantial proportion of the global disease burden resulting from dengue, with 7.5 million apparent cases annually, and possibly more than 30 million infections overall (almost one-tenth of the total number of cases globally) [25]. During my one visit to Jakarta during the late 1990s, I learned that at certain times of the year, the children's wards at area hospitals can be completely full with dengue-infected children, some with the dreaded hemorrhagic complications of the disease or dengue shock syndrome. According to Brandeis University's Donald Shepard, dengue also inflicts tremendous economic costs on Indonesia [26], so this disease helps to keep populations mired in poverty. In response, the Indonesian government is actively working to clear mosquito breeding sites and is actively prioritizing dengue control [21].

Indonesia suffers from one of the worst dengue fever problems globally.

Indonesia is a "classic" blue marble health country because it is a nation with great economic potential that is being held back by widespread helminth infections, especially intestinal helminth infections and LF, yaws, leprosy, and dengue fever. It would be of great interest to determine the gains in economic productivity yielded by controlling these diseases, and in the cases of LF, yaws, and leprosy, one day actually eliminating them.

Japan

In contrast to Indonesia or southwestern China, where NTDs remain widespread, the situation in Japan is almost completely the opposite. Today, intestinal helminth infections, LF, and schistosomiasis—each major components of the worm index of human development—have practically disappeared in Japan, along with many other poverty-related infectious diseases. The story of how NTDs and related diseases were eliminated from Japan, mostly in the three decades following World War II, is an important story, and an instructive one.

By the end of the war, the Japanese economy was in a state of ruin, as was its health-care infrastructure. Poverty was rampant, and Japan was for all practical purposes an impoverished developing nation. Infant and maternal mortality rates had skyrocketed, and tuberculosis was reported to be the leading cause of death [27]. Moreover, malaria, cholera, smallpox, and trachoma were endemic, while in 1948 a new form of scrub typhus had emerged known as Tsutsugamushi disease [27]. Just as in southwestern China, where today human feces are still used as an agricultural fertilizer, thereby helping to promote soilborne intestinal helminth infections, so too was the case in Japan [27]. Indeed, a 1949 nationwide study of intestinal parasites based on fecal examinations revealed that the prevalence of both intestinal roundworm and whipworm exceeded 60%, although the rates of hookworm infection were surprisingly low—below 5% [27]. LF was endemic, especially in southern Japan, and Asian schistosomiasis was found in several regions, including Katayama (a district of Hiroshima prefecture) and Kyushu in southern Japan.

Over the next two decades, NTD rates fell dramatically, and most were eliminated. The forces responsible for Japan's success in eliminating NTDs have been the subject of much discussion, but for me it comes down to two key factors. First, beginning in the 1960s, Japan experienced explosive economic growth. Together, economic development and urbanization represent two of the most powerful social elements responsible for melting away NTDs and other tropical infections. For example, the medical historian Margaret Humphreys traces the disappearance of malaria in the US South (and I think other tropical infections as well) during the 1930s to New Deal legislation introduced by President Franklin Roosevelt [28]. Among other things, the New Deal was an economic stimulus package that helped transform the United States from an agrarian economy to an industrial one and successfully transplanted farmworkers to factories [28]. Similar dramatic economic improvements in eastern China were, I believe, responsible for equally important reductions in NTDs beginning in the 1980s [29], and help to explain why with respect to NTDs we have an east-west Chinese poverty and NTD gradient, as highlighted above.

Postwar school-based deworming was successful in Japan because hookworm did not need to be targeted and because of parallel programs growing out of economic development to prevent post-treatment reinfection.

A second critical factor was the establishment of a nongovernmental organization known as the Japanese Association of Parasite Control (JPAC), which implemented school-based deworming in order to reduce ascariasis and trichuriasis infection rates [30]. JPAC was integrated with family planning organizations in order to develop school-based programs. School-based deworming is especially useful for ascariasis and trichuriasis because epidemiological and mathematical modeling studies show that children living in endemic areas harbor the largest numbers of *Ascaris* and *Trichuris* worms, so that targeting children could dramatically reduce the number of parasite eggs in the environment and ultimately interrupt transmission. This situation contrasts with hookworm infection, where both children and adults (including women of reproductive age) often experience moderate and heavy infections. Moreover, single-dose deworming medicine is often less effective for treating hookworm infection than ascariasis. Because the prevalence of hookworm infection was low in Japan even in the years immediately following the war [27], it was possible to focus deworming only on the elimination of ascariasis and trichuriasis.

Similarly, Asian schistososomiasis disappeared from Japan through targeted treatment of infected individuals, together with environmental control aimed at molluscan intermediate hosts and pouring concrete into snail wetland habitats [30]. LF elimination efforts began in 1962 and were focused in Okinawa and elsewhere in the southern part of the country, where *W. bancrofti* was the overwhelming filarial species [31]. The major approaches to LF control included mass screening by looking for microfilariae in the blood, followed by treatment with diethylcarbamazine citrate (DEC), together with insecticidal spraying of dichlorodiphenyltrichloroethane (DDT) or malathion to destroy the mosquito vector intermediate hosts [31]. The infection rates subsequently fell to near zero by 1971, and LF was declared eliminated from Japan in 1978 [31]. DDT application through residual spraying was also instrumental in Japan's efforts to eliminate malaria, along with expanded use of antimalarial drugs, swamp drainage, and ecological management of rice paddies and farms [27].

I believe that NTD elimination efforts through MDA work best when parallel efforts are in place to economically develop and urbanize the region or the nation. The synergy derived from these approaches can rapidly and profoundly reduce the prevalence of these diseases. Exactly why economic development and urbanization have such a powerful impact is still not well elucidated. Clearly, such social determinants are linked to sanitary disposal of human waste that can help to interrupt intestinal helminth and schistosome life cycles. Economic improvements also allow for better or more efficient implementation of environmental control measures such as swamp drainage and ecological management of farms and livestock. In addition, leaving farms and entering factories can help reduce people's exposure to insect vectors that might transmit LF or malaria. For example, Margaret Humphreys has noted that these factors linked to urbanization were partly responsible for the disappearance of malaria and other neglected diseases (including some NTDs) beginning with Franklin Roosevelt's New Deal legislation during the 1930s [28].

> *Economic development and urbanization are powerful social forces that reduce the prevalence and intensity of NTDs.*

South Korea

The story of endemic NTDs in South Korea, especially intestinal helminth infections, bears many similarities to that of postwar Japan. In the years following the signing of the Korean Armistice Agreement, which established the Korean Demilitarized Zone in 1953, South Korea (the Republic of Korea) suffered from high rates of poverty and poverty-related diseases, including tuberculosis, malaria, and intestinal helminth infections. In response, programs for family planning and the elimination of tuberculosis were launched, and a Korea Association for Parasite Eradication (KAPE) was established in 1964 to conduct mass fecal examinations on the population and twice yearly deworming [32]. Also (and as in Japan), the Korean economy grew almost exponentially, from a GDP of approximately $30 billion in 1960 to well more than $1 trillion over the ensuing 50 years. Such explosive postwar economic growth, together with aggressive urbanization, modernization, and technological innovation, is sometimes referred to as the "miracle on the Han River."

As in Japan, postwar economic development was an important driving force for reducing NTDs, along with a highly committed Korea Association for Parasite Eradication.

Through a KAPE-led implementation of twice-yearly deworming and parallel legislative support known as the Parasitic Disease Prevention Act, the national prevalence rates of ascariasis fell dramatically—from 55% in 1969 to around 10% by 1980, and then to almost zero by 1990 [32]. Following the elimination of ascariasis, KAPE was reorganized as a nongovernmental organization known as the Korean Association of Health Promotion [32]. However, while intestinal helminth infections have disappeared, two foodborne trematodiases transmitted by eating uncooked fish—clonorchiasis and metagonimiasis—remain extant as important zoonotic and helminthic NTDs [32]. And vivax malaria has also been reintroduced into South Korea from the North [33].

In some respects, the NTD situation in North Korea today resembles South Korea's NTD problem in the immediate postwar years.

In contrast to South Korea, North Korea's economy has not progressed significantly since 1953, so the NTD situation in the Democratic People's Republic of Korea somewhat resembles that of the Republic of Korea in the years immediately following the 1953 armistice. In addition to vivax malaria, it is not surprising that intestinal helminth infections [34], foodborne trematodiases [35], malnutrition [36], and tuberculosis [37] remain widespread.

Summary Points

1. MDA is most effective when it occurs along with aggressive economic development.
2. Following the end of World War II and the Korean War, Japan and South Korea, respectively, experienced explosive economic and industrial growth, together with urbanization. These forces in concert with MDA led to the elimination of several important poverty-promoting NTDs, including intestinal helminth infections, LF, and schistosomiasis.
3. Similar explosive economic growth beginning in the 1980s helped to facilitate NTD control in eastern China. However, southwestern China has been left behind, and widespread poverty and NTDs remain in that region.
4. NTDs also remain widespread in Indonesia, where MDA treatment coverage reaches only a small part of its population at risk for NTDs.
5. Together, southwestern China and Indonesia constitute of the global "hotspots" for NTDs [38].

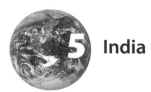 **5 India**

With almost 1.3 billion people, India has the world's second-largest population, but it is projected to overtake China in the coming years. India also has a large economy, with a GDP of almost $2 trillion, ranked eleventh among the G20 nations and the European Union. However, there is room and promise for enormous economic growth, with some projections indicating that by the year 2035, the size of India's economy might be exceeded only by the United States and China [1]. Included among the major sectors of this economic growth are agricultural production (currently India ranks second worldwide in this category); industry (fossil fuels and energy, engineering, pharmaceuticals, mining, and textiles); and information technology [1].

While India has tremendous economic potential, it still has three-quarters of a billion people who live on less than $2 per day and 300 million who live on essentially no money.

Then there is the hidden and largely forgotten India. The country hosts a crushing level of poverty, with approximately one-quarter of its population—roughly 300 million people—who live on virtually nothing, that is, below the 2005–14 World Bank poverty figure of $1.25 per day [2]. More than one-half of the population—almost 750 million people—lives on less than $2 per day [3]. Although poverty is widespread and even pervasive in India [4], as noted in chapter 3, it is particularly severe in the northeastern parts of the country, especially in states such as Bihar, Uttar Pradesh, and Orissa, as well as in Assam [5]. It has also been noted that poverty in India sorts out along a rural versus urban divide [1], although certainly there is also horrific poverty in India's urban slums. Such profound poverty, together with explosive population growth, may threaten India's future economic growth [1].

Overview of India's NTDs

NTDs flourish in the midst of India's rural poverty [4]. Despite its economic potential, India has the sixth-highest worm index of any of the G20 nations, with some of the largest numbers of people living with intestinal helminth infections or LF anywhere in the world [6]. Malnutrition is also pervasive in India, in part because of the widespread prevalence of intestinal helminth infections, together with intestinal protozoan infections and diarrheal diseases (including rotavirus and bacterial gastrointestinal infections). Shown in table 5.1 is an earlier analysis from 2011 of the major NTDs in India [4], when we estimated that there were almost 285 million cases of ascariasis,

Table 5.1. The major NTDs in India and South Asia, ranked by prevalence

Disease	Number of cases in India (% of global disease burden)	Number of cases in India and South Asia (% of global disease burden)	Estimated number of DALYs in South Asia
Ascariasis	140 million (17%)	237 million (29%)	0.4–3.0 million
Trichuriasis	73 million (12%)	147 million (24%)	0.5–1.5 million
Hookworm infection	71 million (12%)	130 million (23%)	0.6–5.6 million
Lymphatic filariasis	<6 million (5%) (based on 0.53% prevalence)	<60 million (50%)	2.9 million
Trachoma	1 million (1%–2%)	2 million (2%–4%)	<0.1 million
Visceral leishmaniasis	Not determined	200,000–300,000 cases (40%–60%)	0.4–1.0 million
Leprosy	87,190 registered cases (41%)	120,456 registered cases (57%)c	0.1 million
Rabies	20,000 cases/deaths (36%)	≥20,000 cases/deaths (>36%)	Not determined
Japanese encephalitis	1,500–4,000 (incidence)	1,000–3,000 (incidence: Nepal); 100–200 (incidence: Sri Lanka)	0.3 million
Dengue	Not determined	Not determined	0.4 million
Total			5.6–14.8 million

Source: [4], doi:10.1371/journal.pntd.0001222.t002.

trichuriasis, and hookworm infection in that country. Beyond these intestinal helminth infections and LF, the major illnesses also include leprosy, kala-azar (visceral leishmaniasis), dengue fever and other arboviral infections, rabies, snake envenomation, cholera, and other diarrheal diseases. In addition, although they are not classified as NTDs, falciparum malaria and tuberculosis both also represent important neglected diseases in India.

Intestinal Helminth Infections

India has the world's largest number of people, especially children and women of reproductive age, suffering from ascariasis, trichuriasis, and hookworm infection. These intestinal helminth infections have plagued India since ancient times, and even Mohandas Gandhi was said to suffer from hookworm infection toward the end of his life [7]. According to WHO's PCT database, India has more than 200 million children who require frequent and regular deworming for their intestinal helminth infections [8]. However, India's most impoverished northeast region likely suffers from the highest prevalence rates. According to one recent study, the overall prevalence of intestinal helminth infections among children living in Bihar state is 68%, led by ascariasis and hookworm infection. Many of Bihar's children routinely practice open defecation and cleanse their hands with soil. Low maternal literacy has also been linked to high rates of infection [9].

India has the world's largest number of children living with worms in their intestines.

Intestinal helminth infections are preventing a generation of children in India from achieving their full intellectual, cognitive, and economic potential.

Such high prevalence rates justify the need to practice mass drug administration (MDA) for intestinal helminth infections using once- or twice-yearly deworming medicines, because of their positive impact on pediatric nutrition and cognition. For instance, in the slums of Lucknow (located in Uttar Pradesh), it was found that twice-yearly deworming with albendazole resulted in significant weight gain among malnourished children. Specifically, the treated children gained an extra kilogram in weight compared with untreated children in neighboring slums [10]. Despite such successes, according to WHO, only 15.7% of India's school-age children and 7.5% of preschool-age children who require deworming actually receive medication [8]. Therefore, there is an urgent need for the government of India to expand its deworming coverage.

The Stigmatizing NTDs: LF and Leprosy

India is equally affected by lymphatic filariasis (LF), a highly disfiguring and stigmatizing condition caused by the filarial parasite, *Wuchereria bancrofti* and transmitted by *Culex* mosquitoes. India suffers from the largest number of people affected by LF and requiring MDA. According to WHO data for the year 2013, almost 500 million people in India require annual MDA with a combination of DEC and albendazole, or roughly 40% of the world's population requiring treatment for LF [11]. In its most advanced form, LF causes obstruction of the lymphatics that over time can lead to disfigurement and distortion of the lower limbs and breasts, while LF-induced hydrocele affects the male genitals (fig. 5.1). Thus, beyond its health effects, LF is notorious for its impact on India's socioeconomic development.

Figure 5.1.
Lymphedema of the lower extremities is one of the advanced clinical manifestations of lymphatic filariasis. Courtesy of Vivek Singh / Global Assignment by Getty Images. All rights reserved.

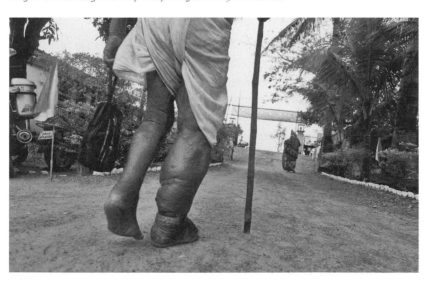

Social scientists have undertaken studies to evaluate the full impact of LF. In 2000, when the Millennial Development Goals were launched, it was determined that LF cost India hundreds of millions of dollars annually in lost work productivity and health-care costs [12]. Somewhat less quantifiable but equally important is the misery and poor quality of life for people living in India with LF. One recent and sobering study is the consequence of LF hydrocele on human sexual and marital life in Orissa, which reveals nearly 100% dissatisfaction or incapacity in sexual relations, with resulting deterioration in the marriage. According to this study, led by a social and behavioral research unit of the Indian Council of Medical

LF is a leading cause of social stigma and isolation in India.

Research, an LF hydrocele patient is considered a last choice for marriage in Orissa [13].

Today MDA is conducted in India in collaboration with the Global Programme to Eliminate LF (GPELF) to reduce the burden and ultimately eliminate the disease. MDA, when implemented over consecutive years, has been shown to actually interrupt transmission of LF, because it targets the microfilarial stages in the blood that are taken up by mosquitoes. When MDA coverage reaches a certain level, there are not sufficient microfilariae circulating among the population, so the transmission of the disease halts and LF can be eliminated. The worldwide impact of GPELF has been impressive. Launched in 2000, its activities have helped to provide more than 6 billion treatments, resulting in the prevention of almost 100 million LF cases, including an estimated 19 million hydrocele cases [14]. India's health and economy has greatly benefited from this activity [15]. In 2013, WHO estimated that approximately one-half of India's eligible population has received MDA for LF [11]. In addition to MDA, there is a parallel commitment from both GPELF and the Indian government for managing the morbidities linked to LF lymphedema and hydrocele [16, 17]. Community-led initiatives, including faith-based programs, are instrumental in lymphedema and hydrocele management [17].

India also accounts for almost one-half of the world's cases of another highly disfiguring and stigmatizing NTD—leprosy [18]. Based partly on ancient texts dating back to 2000 BC, leprosy is believed to have originated in India before spreading along trade routes (or through human migrations linked to war) eastward to China and westward to the Middle East, Africa, and Europe, before its transatlantic passage to the New World [19]. The stigma from disfigurement and fear of contracting leprosy also began in ancient times and was even noted by early European colonialists to lead to ritualistic suicide [19]. According to Drs. Jesse Jacob and Carlos Franco-Paredes in a 2008 article in *PLOS NTDs*, in an effort to destigmatize leprosy, Gandhi made the unprecedented gesture of inviting a noted Sanskrit scholar who suffered from the disease, Parchure Shastri, to his ashram in 1939 in order to provide care, change his wound dressings, and provide daily foot massages. Ultimately, an image of Gandhi tending to the scholar was placed on a national postage stamp with the words "leprosy is curable" [19].

In 1955, a national control program was formed that gained momentum in the 1980s when a multidrug therapy became available for large populations. Through this approach, by 2005 the number of cases in India was reduced to less than 1 case per 10,000 people—a target set for leprosy elimination at the national level [19]. However, in some poor rural areas, the number of leprosy cases remains high [19], and as noted above, India accounts for one-half of leprosy cases globally.

"END 7"

In 2006 at the Clinton Global Initiative, together with colleagues I helped to create a Global Network for NTDs in order to raise awareness and mobilize resources for MDA and other control and elimination measures [20]. One of our signature campaigns is an "END 7" operation focused on linking MDA for up to seven NTDs—ascariasis, trichuriasis, hookworm infection, LF, onchocerciasis, schistosomiasis, and trachoma (http://www.END7.org). Previously under the direction of Dr. Neeraj Mistry, a key target area for NTD advocacy is the nation of India, with a focus on intestinal helminth infections and LF [21]. Through support from the Bill & Melinda Gates Foundation, the Global Network for NTDs and its END 7 campaign are working in collaboration with the Indian government to expand its MDA efforts, especially in remote and marginalized communities. These efforts include a national roadmap for the elimination of LF. In order to further destigmatize the NTDs and to promote community acceptance of those suffering from these illnesses, the Global Network for NTDs appointed Bollywood star Abhishek Bachchan as its global ambassador for India.

According to Nandini Pillai and Shailesh Vaite, who directed Global Network for NTD operations in India, the nation is beginning to make signifi-

cant progress against both LF and intestinal helminth infections. With regard to LF, the population requiring treatment has begun to drop and will
continue to fall as Indian government experts proceed with their monitoring
and evaluation efforts in order to verify the interruption of transmission.
One of the biggest challenges to LF elimination in India has been high levels
of transmission occurring in 31 "hotspot" districts. These hotspot areas are
mostly extremely remote and rural areas, or in some cases
they are politically complex. The Indian government is now
redoubling its commitment to such districts, with plans to
implement two MDAs per year. For intestinal helminth infections, it has launched an annual "National Deworming
Day" for children under the age of 19. During India's first
National Deworming Day, an estimated 89 million children in 11 states received MDA.

Given its modest costs and significant health and economic impact, MDA for LF and intestinal helminth infections represents one of the greatest returns on investment for the nation of India.

Beyond the complicated logistics of providing MDA
for vast numbers of people in remote, rural areas is the
problem of coordinating monitoring and surveillance activities, and making sufficient funds available at the federal level of the Indian government. Although the costs for providing MDA
are extremely modest, often pennies a person, when multiplied by the hundreds of millions of people who require MDA in a nation like the India, the
price nonetheless runs in the millions of dollars. Still, this is a nation that
likely spends many times more annually on developing and maintaining a
nuclear stockpile or other less essential items. LF and intestinal helminth
infections are a major reason why India's bottom 750 million people cannot
achieve their full physical and intellectual potential or escape poverty. There
may be no greater return on investment than MDA activities that target
helminth infections.

The Vector-Borne NTDs: Kala-Azar (Visceral Leishmaniasis), Malaria, and Dengue Fever

The problem of NTDs in India extends well beyond worm infections. Among
the most serious NTDs are those that are transmitted by insect vectors. LF
is a helminth infection transmitted by mosquitoes, but other diseases transmitted by insects include kala-azar (visceral leishmaniasis) and malaria, as

well as dengue and other arboviruses [22]. India today accounts for most of the world's kala-azar and a substantial portion of the global burden of disease from malaria and dengue.

World Health Day 2014 focused global awareness on the plight of people living in extreme poverty who disproportionately suffer from such vector-borne diseases [23]. Today, as many people die annually from vector-borne diseases as from HIV/AIDS. India's extreme poverty partly accounts for its widespread vector-borne diseases, but for reasons that are still not well established. Poor quality housing without window screens and air conditioning undoubtedly plays an important role, as does inadequate refuse collection, which allows insects to proliferate. Global climate change and its connection to flooding and warmer temperatures are also expected to further promote the emergence of these diseases in India in the coming decades [24].

Kala-azar (visceral leishmaniasis). One of the most important vector-borne NTDs is visceral leishmaniasis, caused by *Leishmania donovani*, also called kala-azar. Transmitted by *Phlebotomus* sandflies, kala-azar is a parasitic infection caused by protozoa that live inside our macrophages—a type of critically important cell of our immune system that ordinarily ingests and destroys invading pathogens that cause infections, such as bacteria. The protozoa parasites that cause kala-azar have evolved to survive and replicate inside macrophages to ultimately cause a severe and highly lethal illness in people that resembles leukemia or lymphoma. Today Bihar, in addition to being "ground zero" for intestinal helminth infections, also hosts the largest concentration of kala-azar cases.

Bihar State in India is "ground zero" for the global kala-azar (visceral leishmaniasis) problem.

Indeed, India alone is believed to account for approximately 60% of the world's kala-azar cases [25], with three-quarters of those occurring among people living in Bihar [26]. Compounding the problem are kala-azar and HIV coinfections, associated with more rapid disease progression and mortality. Moreover, in India underlying malnourishment and nutritional deficiencies are common, and these can exacerbate the disease, while kala-azar itself can cause a severe wasting syndrome sometimes also known as cachexia [27].

Still another major problem facing kala-azar patients in Bihar is access to essential medicines. One of the most effective is a drug initially developed to treat severe fungal infections in the United States and elsewhere and known as liposomal amphotericin B (AmBisome). The medicine has to be given in a hospital setting and is administered intravenously over a period of 4 to 10 days. Recently, Médecins Sans Frontières (MSF) and the Rajendra Memorial Research Institute reported success in treating kala-azar patients in a hospital in Bihar with AmBisome, which is produced by the US-based Gilead Sciences [26]. However, delivering AmBisome to large numbers of kala-azar sufferers presents a number of challenges, including the need to improve Bihar's health infrastructure for delivering an intravenous infusion and the maintenance of a temperature-controlled supply chain for the drug [26].

Another factor has been cost. In 2011, Gilead announced that it would partner with WHO to donate almost 500,000 vials for treating more than 50,000 patients over a period of five years [28], but MSF has responded that "it can not be seen as a global solution as it only covers a small proportion of patients worldwide. We have doubts about whether this is a sustainable solution: more needs to be done to ensure treatment is affordable and available worldwide in the long-term, and that means encouraging competition from similar products to bring down the price of treatment" [29]. As an alternative, an indigenous preparation—Fungisome—has become available in India and may also be effective for the treatment of kala-azar [30].

There is the potential to eliminate kala-azar in Bihar and India. The twin pillars of an elimination strategy include case detection and treatment with AmBisome or Fungisome, as well as other medication, together with insecticidal spraying to destroy *Phlebotomus* sandflies. The mainstay of sandfly vector control has been indoor residual spraying with compounds containing dichlorodiphenyltrichloroethane (DDT). However, in studies led by the Liverpool School of Tropical Medicine in collaboration with the Indian Council of Medical Research, it has been recently noted that indoor residual spraying has not been consistently applied and sandfly resistance to DDT has emerged. In its place, it has been recommended to substitute pyrethroid insecticides for DDT [31]. Doing so would also avoid the potential environmental consequences of widespread DDT use.

Malaria. Increasing evidence also points to a huge burden of disease and mortality from malaria. Transmitted by *Anopheles* mosquitoes, two major forms of the disease plague India: falciparum malaria is associated with high mortality, and vivax malaria is linked to severe disability. Revised estimates from the Million Death Study Collaborators—a group that seeks to better understand causes of death in rural India, where people often die outside of health facilities and without autopsies, have determined that 1.3 million deaths associated with fever occur in rural India annually, of which an astonishing 205,000 deaths before the age of 70 are due to malaria [32]. Additional estimates indicate that India alone accounts for 35% of the world's malaria cases [33].

Malaria has emerged as a leading killer in India.

Dengue. A dengue fever epidemic of huge proportions is simultaneously emerging in India. By some accounts, we are in the midst of a global dengue pandemic, with almost 100 million new cases occurring in the year 2013—and approximately one-third of those cases occur in India [34]. Dengue is associated with high fever, vomiting, severe headache, skin rash, and severe joint pains known as "breakbone fever." It can also result in bleeding and shock leading to death in some patients. The most efficient mosquito vector for transmitting dengue is the urban-dwelling *Aedes aegypti* mosquito. New Delhi and other localities in India have experienced dramatic epidemics that overrun hospitals [35]. Some estimates indicate that 37 million dengue infections occur annually, with more than 200,000 hospitalizations [35]. However, the vast majority of India's cases are either undiagnosed or underreported, owing in part to governmental failure to implement a dengue surveillance system. According to Gardiner Harris, then a *New York Times* India correspondent, dengue is "politically damaging," so some government officials refuse to address the problem, even though some experts indicate that getting infected with dengue fever while living in India is practically inevitable [35]. Whereas kala-azar and malaria are found primarily in rural India, dengue's emergence can be partly attributed to rapid (and disorganized) urbanization in India's massive cities. Indeed, although most NTDs are endemic in poor rural areas and urbanization is in

India's urban areas are in the midst of an alarming and vast dengue epidemic.

many cases linked to reductions in NTDs, with dengue (and a few other diseases) things are different. As noted above, this observation is mostly due to the fact that its chief vector, *Ae. aegypti*, is found predominantly in degraded urban areas.

To date, success in the control of all three major vector-borne diseases by targeting mosquitoes (LF, malaria, and dengue) and sandflies (kala-azar) has been elusive. Except for LF, there are no MDA approaches for these diseases. Instead, there is an urgent need for increased engagement by village-level health-care workers in the matters of early detection and treatment, as well as for increased resources for strengthening patient management and vector control [36]. Ultimately, new vaccines to prevent malaria, dengue, and kala-azar, as well as hookworm infection, would constitute important new biotechnologies for control and elimination. Later, we will see and try to better understand some of the socioeconomic challenges to developing vaccines that target poverty-related diseases.

Other Neglected Diseases and the NCDs

Aside from helminth infections and vector-borne infections, India accounts for approximately one-third of the annual 55,000–70,000 global deaths from rabies, mostly canine rabies [37]; an estimated 45,900 annual deaths from snake envenomation, especially from the spectacled cobra, common krait, saw-scaled viper, and Russell's viper [38]; and thousands of deaths annually from cholera and other neglected diarrheal diseases [39]. India also accounts for almost one-quarter of the world's tuberculosis cases, 6% of the 35 million people worldwide living with HIV/AIDS, and 15% of the global deaths from NCDs [33, 40].

Increasingly, we are seeing NTDs superimposed on co-endemic NCDs among India's poor.

As NCDs increase among the poor in G20 nations such as India, we are beginning to see some interesting comorbidities among people with both neglected infectious diseases and NCDs. A good example is India's tuberculosis and diabetes mellitus co-epidemic [41]. The prevalence of type 2 diabetes is believed to be rising at "alarming" rates in India, and the Indian government is responding through programs of increased screening and testing [42]. Among tuberculosis patients, the prevalence of diabetes appears to be especially high. In one community-based study, the prevalence of diabetes was 29% among tuberculosis patients and was significantly associated with tuberculosis microorganisms in the sputum [43]. Still another example is the effect of dengue on people with diabetes or hypertension. It was shown in Kerala State, for instance, that the mortality from dengue was far higher in adults with these underlying noncommunicable diseases [44]. Accordingly, there have been calls for joint approaches that integrate neglected and noncommunicable diseases in India [45].

Concluding Remarks

Together with greater resources devoted to strengthened health systems, in a 2011 interview in one of India's large newspapers, the *Hindu*, I pointed out how the country has an extraordinary scientific infrastructure for building new technologies to combat its heavy disease burden from NTDs and other poverty-related diseases [46]. I have also highlighted how many of these resources have been inappropriately diverted to other activities. For example, in a 2010 *PLOS NTDs* article, "Nuclear Weapons and Neglected Diseases: The 'Ten-Thousand-to-One Gap,'" I estimated that globally the world spends 10,000 times more on developing, stockpiling, and maintaining nuclear weapons than it does on its neglected diseases [47]. India is a prime example, as at that time it had in hand between 75 and 110 nuclear weapons [47]. The good news is that there is increasing awareness by government leaders that India's economic future is actually being held back by vast numbers of people living with NTDs. NTD control and elimination is in many cases relatively inexpensive and could provide huge investment returns.

Summary Points

1. India has approximately 300 million people who live on virtually no income—below the previous World Bank poverty figure of $1.25 per day—and 750 million people living on less than $2 per day. India's extreme poverty disproportionately occurs among its northeastern states, for example, in Bihar, Uttar Pradesh, and Orissa, as well as in Assam.

2. NTDs are having a profound health and economic impact on India's bottom economic segments, and there is much to be done. For example, more than 200 million Indian schoolchildren require deworming, and yet according to WHO, only a small percentage of them have access to regular deworming medicines.

3. LF is also a major cause of socioeconomic underdevelopment, as well as social stigma in India. Approximately one-half of India's eligible population receives MDA annually. If this proportion were immediately expanded, India could potentially eliminate LF by the

year 2020. The Global Network for NTDs, together with the Indian government and Bollywood star Abhishek Bachchan, is working to raise awareness about intestinal helminth infections and LF and the opportunities for MDA. A major focus includes intensified MDA in highly endemic "hotspot" districts and National Deworming Days.

4. Vector-borne tropical infections are equally widespread. The most devastating in terms of morbidity and mortality are kala-azar (*Phlebotomus* sandflies), malaria (*Anopheles* mosquitoes), and dengue fever (*Aedes* mosquitoes).

    a. Bihar state in India may have the world's largest number of cases of kala-azar. There is an urgent need to expand case detection and treatment efforts using commercially available liposomal amphotericin B (AmBisome) or an indigenous equivalent, and to improve vector control through insecticidal spraying. DDT resistance may necessitate greater use of pyrethroid insecticides.

    b. More than 200,000 people in India die annually from malaria before the age of 70. Most of these deaths occur in rural areas.

    c. Dengue is sweeping through India's major urban centers. More than 30 million incident (new) infections occur annually.

5. Canine rabies, snake envenomation, and diarrheal diseases (including cholera) represent additional important causes of NTD-linked morbidities and mortalities.

6. As NCDs rise in India, we are now seeing co-epidemics of neglected diseases and NCDs. Important examples are the high rates of type 2 diabetes patients with either tuberculosis or dengue.

7. There are urgent needs for the Indian government to take greater action to combat its own NTDs and to expand its biotechnology infrastructure in order to focus on these diseases.

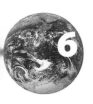

6 Sub-Saharan Africa

Nigeria and South Africa

The NTDs were conceived in the years following the launch of the Millennial Development Goals as part of a pro-poor strategy for Africa, with a focus on seven high-prevalence diseases that could be targeted with a "rapid impact" package of donated medicines [1]. Today, programs of mass drug administration are under way in more than 20 sub-Saharan African countries, led by USAID and British DFID NTD programs, with additional support from a private END Fund. In 2015, WHO determined that 35% of the eligible population in its African region is receiving access to essential NTD medicines [2]. In all, 229.5 million people in sub-Saharan Africa received treatment in 2013 [2]. Over a similar time frame following the launch of the MDGs, the World Bank estimates that Africa's economy has grown by an average of 4.4% annually [3]. This rate of growth in Africa has had a steep trajectory and may now even exceed Asia's economic growth, which some experts have suggested has been comparatively flat overall [4].

Since the launch of PEPFAR, PMI, GFATM, and the USAID and DFID NTD Programs, some countries in sub-Saharan Africa have experienced impressive economic growth.

Based on the inverse association between national human development indices and worm indices noted previously, it would be useful to learn how much of Africa's economic improvement might have resulted from the African component of the reductions in new HIV/AIDS, TB, and malaria cases, or the 25–39% decrease in global prevalence of some major NTDs such as LF, trachoma, onchocerciasis, and ascariasis—results that as I pointed out earlier were determined from the Global Disease Burden Study 2013.

Despite sub-Saharan Africa's impressive economic gains, one-half the region still lives with essentially no income.

While Africa's health and economic gains are impressive, their rise over the past decade continues to leave behind the massive yet forgotten bottom segment that remains mired in extreme poverty. The World Bank estimates that in 2011, 46.8% of sub-Saharan Africa's population lived on less than $1.25 per day [5]. In some nations, such as Madagascar, almost 90% of the population lives below this World Bank poverty level [6].

The Potent Forces of Poverty and Conflict

Sub-Saharan Africa's conflict and postconflict countries, such as South Sudan and Central African Republic, are especially vulnerable to NTDs, as armed struggle is a potent force that depletes health systems already weakened from decades of profound poverty. As a result, the conflict and postconflict nations in Africa suffer from the world's highest rates of NTDs [7]. In some areas of South Sudan, trachoma, schistosomiasis, and LF are actually hyperendemic [7], meaning there is a constantly high prevalence or incidence of these NTDs. Other important examples of poverty and NTDs in postconflict Africa are offered by the three countries most affected by Ebola virus infection in 2014–15: Guinea, Liberia, and Sierra Leone. These countries have emerged only relatively recently out of conflict and suffer from enormously high rates of extreme poverty and NTDs.

Conflict combines with poverty to promote NTD hyperendemicity.

While today Ebola virus infection is the best-known NTD linked to the conflicts in West Africa, it is also far less common than other diseases. Shown in table 6.1 is a 2015 analysis I published in *PLOS NTDs* indicating that while only about 0.1% of the population was infected with Ebola virus during the epidemic, approximately one-half of the people of Guinea, Liberia, and Sierra Leone suffer from schistosomiasis, hookworm infection, and malaria, as well as highly endemic dengue and onchocerciasis [8]. Together, these diseases combine to produce severe and long-lasting effects from anemia [9], including adverse pregnancy outcomes, reduced worker productivity, and impaired child development [10], such that the NTDs are major contributors to trapping generations of people in poverty.

Table 6.1. Neglected tropical diseases in the three Ebola-affected countries of West Africa

Disease or category	Guinea	Liberia	Sierra Leone	All three countries
Population	12.0 million	4.4 million	6.2 million	22.6 million
Ebola virus infections (as of June 1, 2015)	3,653	12,816	10,666	27,135
Hookworm infection (children)	0.99 million	0.31 million	0.84 million	2.14 million
Ascariasis (children)	0.17 million	0.12 million	0.15 million	0.44 million
Trichuriasis (children)	0.08 million	0.09 million	0.06 million	0.23 million
Schistosomiasis (population requiring MDA in 2013)	2.11 million	1.07 million	1.47 million	4.65 million
Lymphatic filariasis (% of population requiring preventive chemotherapy in 2013)	0.06 million (0.4885%)	0.01 million (0.2366%)	0.03 million (0.5492%)	0.10 million
Onchocerciasis (estimated total population at risk in 2013)	3.28 million	3.09 million	3.18 million	9.55 million
Malaria (reported or confirmed cases)	0.21 million	1.24 million	1.70 million	3.15 million
Dengue (apparent cases)	0.19 million	0.10 million	0.14 million	0.43 million

Source: [8], doi:10.1371/journal.pntd.0003671.t001.

At the height of the Ebola virus crisis in the fall of 2014, I was interviewed almost daily on MSNBC, Fox News, or Bloomberg TV. While it was exciting to speak to large audiences about Ebola virus infection, for me it was also a source of frustration that many anchors and producers on those news shows did not care very much about West Africa's high prevalence NTDs, such as schistosomiasis and hookworm infection, even though in the long run these may represent real disease forces that have been holding back future progress in Guinea, Liberia, and Sierra Leone. In many respects (and with some important exceptions), it is the widespread, nonlethal, debilitating NTDs rather than the relatively rare killer NTDs that truly devastate populations.

The widespread, nonlethal, debilitating NTDs rather than the relatively rare killer NTDs are the ones that truly devastate populations.

Nigeria

With a GDP of more than $0.5 trillion, Nigeria boasts the largest economy in sub-Saharan Africa [11, 12]. Historically, much of the nation's economic engine derives from oil and energy—Nigeria is Africa's largest producer of petroleum, mostly from its oil-rich southern Niger Delta. Despite recent drops in global oil prices that could threaten its economy in the coming years, some of Nigeria's other sectors continue to grow, including agriculture, information technology, telecommunications, and even a thriving and robust motion picture industry [11, 12]. Through diversification, Nigeria's GDP has continued to grow at 6–7% annually over the past two years [11]. Living and working in Houston, Texas, I cannot help but notice the parallels between my city and Lagos, Nigeria's most populated metropolitan area, with more than 20 million people. Both are port cities—Houston on the Gulf of Mexico and Nigeria on the Gulf of Guinea—with massive recent population growth and historical dependence on oil, but also continued economic growth through diversification. It is also ironic that Houston has one of the largest Nigerian expatriate communities in the world. We now have daily nonstop flights to Lagos.

However, as in the other blue marble health countries, Nigeria's massive growth continues to leave a large proportion of the population behind, who struggle with severe poverty and disease. In 2010, the World Bank estimated that 62% of Nigeria's population subsists on less than $1.25 per day [13], with 82% of its population making less than $2 per day [14]. With a total population now estimated at 180 million people, these numbers mean that almost 150 million Nigerians live on practically nothing.

Nigeria is a classic blue marble health country: it boasts 6–7% annual economic growth that leaves behind 150 million people in extreme poverty.

It is no surprise that NTDs flourish amidst widespread poverty. In a *PLOS NTDs* article that I wrote in 2012 with two Nigerian scientists working in Houston at Texas Children's Hospital, we highlighted Nigeria as "ground zero" for the world's high-prevalence NTDs [15]. As shown in table 6.2 taken from that paper, Nigeria ranks first among African nations in terms of the number of people infected with intestinal helminth infections, schistosomiasis, LF, and onchocerciasis [15]. It also ranks first globally in the number of people infected with schistosomiasis and onchocerciasis, third globally for LF cases, and fourth for hookworm infection

Table 6.2. Ranking of Nigeria by neglected tropical disease cases and prevalence

Disease	Estimated number of cases in Nigeria	Ranking in Africa	% of global disease burden	Ranking globally
Ascariasis	55 million	1	7	5 (behind India, Indonesia, China, and Bangladesh)
Hookworm infection	38 million	1	7	Tied for 4 with China (behind India, Indonesia, and Bangladesh)
Trichuriasis	34 million	1	6	4 (behind India, Indonesia, and Bangladesh)
Schistosomiasis	29 million	1	14	1
Lymphatic filariasis	25 million (and 80 million–121 million estimated at risk, requiring MDA)	1	21	3
Onchocerciasis	30 million at risk, requiring MDA	1	36	1
Trachoma	18 million at risk	Not determined	Not determined	Not determined
Leprosy	4,531 (registered prevalence)	4	2	7

Source: [15], doi:10.1371/journal.pntd.0001600.t001.

and trichuriasis [15]. Moreover, based on WHO's PCT data, our calculated worm index for Nigeria is 1.012, ranking it only behind Democratic Republic of Congo as the highest worm index for any of the world's 25 largest nations [16].

How do we reconcile Nigeria's strong economic indicators in the face of terrible poverty and high rates of NTDs? Fundamentally, the numbers mean that, at least in the past, the modest funds required to support MDA are available, particularly since the essential NTD medicines are being donated, but that the Nigerian government has not yet demonstrated the political will needed to expand MDA for its poorest people. For example, according to WHO, less than 20% of the population who require MDA for intestinal helminth infections or LF receive treatment

Nigeria is "ground zero" for Africa's NTDs in the sense that it leads African nations in the number of cases of all three major intestinal helminth infections, schistosomiasis, LF, and onchocerciasis.

annually [17, 18], while only 6% of the population receives access to praziquantel for schistosomiasis [19]. In some cases, Boko Haram activities have prevented government-led MDA efforts in parts of northern Nigeria [20], but this aspect can account for only a small percentage of the low MDA coverage rates.

Only a tiny percentage of Nigeria's population currently receives MDA for NTDs.

To help facilitate MDA activities in Nigeria, the Atlanta-based Carter Center has an active schistosomiasis control program that works with Nigerian health authorities in six states, integrating control with the other major NTDs targeted by the rapid impact package [21]. The Carter Center is also working to expand LF and river blindness elimination efforts and advancing toward guinea worm eradication there [22]. In parallel, USAID and DFID have pooled resources to provide $36 million over four years as support for NTD MDA efforts [23]. An important five-year program known as ENVISION, supported by USAID through RTI International, which works in partnership with eight nongovernmental organizations, including the Carter Center [24], is also contributing to a scale-up of national MDA efforts, while DFID supports an NTD program through the UK-based Sightsavers [25].

Through its Ministry of Health, the government of Nigeria in turn has launched a 2013–17 "Master Plan for NTDs," a five-year implementation plan expected to cost approximately $300 million [26]. Nigeria's health ministry has also shown a level of innovation in terms of its ability to expand treatment coverage. For example, Dr. Jonathan Yisa Jiya, who ran Nigeria's onchocerciasis program, has linked LF with malaria treatment coverage, in light of the fact that both NTDs are transmitted by *Anopheles* mosquitoes in rural areas and can be prevented through use of insecticide-treated nets [27]. Nigeria has been a pioneer in its effort to eliminate polio and could build on this infrastructure to target its NTDs. Indeed this anti-polio infrastructure turned out to be essential in preventing the Ebola virus infection from igniting into an epidemic in Nigeria.

The forces hindering MDA in Nigeria are not unique: complicated logistics, decentralization, inadequate resource allocation, and lack of political will.

Through support of the Bill & Melinda Gates Foundation, the Global Network for NTDs based at the Sabin Vaccine Institute has worked with the Nigerian government to expand awareness for the NTDs across different administrative sectors and to extend its master plan beyond 2017 [28]. However, according to some, the total federal funding that was truly allocated for NTDs by the Nigerian government was only $1.5 million in 2014, and now even this modest amount has been reduced to only $1 million in 2015. Currently, much of the NTD control is placed in the hands of the governors of the many Nigerian states and local health officials. The intent of decentralization is to strengthen primary health care in the individual states and regions. But, as we have seen before in India and will see again in Brazil, this approach often fragments NTD control and elimination efforts, especially in large nations with populations exceeding 100 million people.

We need greater engagement from Nigeria's research institutes and universities to develop and produce innovative solutions for its NTDs.

Unfortunately, Nigeria's research institutes and universities have yet to live up to their potential to expand NTD activities in order to embrace research and development for new technologies. With respect to MDA for NTDs, Nigeria's universities have, like its government, largely underperformed. For example, despite the country's enormous economic capacity, none of Nigeria's universities are ranked among Africa's leading universities, nor are they even listed in the well-recognized QS World University Rankings 2015/16 [29]. Nigeria urgently needs a top-flight research university to help lead innovation for its NTDs.

South Africa

South Africa has the second-largest economy in sub-Saharan Africa and is the continent's only G20 nation. However, of its estimated 53 million people, almost 10% live in extreme poverty [13]. If Nigeria is ground zero for Africa's NTDs, the same might be said of South Africa for its HIV/AIDS epidemic. More than six million people live with HIV/AIDS in South Africa [30], putting the overall national adult prevalence at 19.1% [31]. However, in KwaZulu-Natal on the Indian Ocean coast and near the northern borders with Zimbabwe and Mozambique, the HIV/AIDS prevalence according to some is closer to an astounding 40% [31]. Coinciding with its profound HIV/AIDS epidemic, South Africa also suffers from devastatingly high rates of opportunistic TB [30]. To its credit, the South African government has implemented an ambitious antiretroviral therapy program, the largest in the world according to AVERT, an international AIDS charity based in the

United Kingdom [31]. These national efforts include more than \$1 billion of South African government investments to operate its HIV/AIDS treatment and prevention programs [31].

NTDs are also widespread in South Africa. Approximately 5.3 million people require annual MDA for schistosomiasis [19], and about one-half as many for intestinal helminth infections [17]. Schistosomiasis is probably South Africa's most important NTD, but for reasons that are not immediately appreciated. An emerging body of evidence indicates that schistosomiasis could actually be South Africa's most important cofactor in its HIV/AIDS epidemic, especially in KwaZulu-Natal, where schistosomiasis is widespread and HIV/AIDS prevalence in the highest. The important links between schistosomiasis and HIV/AIDS are worth exploring in detail.

As explained earlier, schistosomiasis is transmitted by snails and is acquired while standing in fresh water teeming with the infective stages of schistosomes—larvae known as cercariae. Chronic schistosomiasis is associated with chronic bladder fibrosis, leading to long-standing damage to the bladder and its associated ureters. Schistosome eggs are carcinogens and cause a unique bladder cancer. Schistosomiasis can also lead to chronic kidney disease and even renal failure and death. Although the South African government has been recognized for its efforts to fight HIV/AIDS, free and donated generic praziquantel, which is available for almost all of sub-Saharan Africa, is—almost inexplicably—not used to treat schistosomiasis in South Africa, whose health administration still requires the use of a purchased commercial brand drug instead [32].

This decision is especially regrettable given findings by the University of Oslo's Dr. Eyrun Kjetland, who has found high rates of female genital schistosomiasis (FGS) in the country. FGS is caused by *Schistosoma haematobium*, the same cause of bladder and kidney disease identified above. It results when the terminal-spine-shaped schistosome eggs are deposited in the uterus, cervix, and lower genital tract of South Africa's girls and women [33]. The lesions cause pain, bleeding, and social stigma leading to depression. Kjetland and her colleagues have also shown that *S. haematobium* is an important cofactor in Africa's AIDS epidemic [33]. Presumably, the ulcerative lesions in the genital tract of South Africa's girls and women offer new routes of entry for the human immunodeficiency virus (HIV). Today, FGS represents one of South Africa's most potent cofactors in its horrific AIDS epidemic. Similar observations have been made by a team at Weil Cornell Medical College led by Dr. Jennifer Downs [34].

FGS is now widespread among girls and young women who live in extreme poverty in KwaZulu-Natal [35]. Working in the Ugu District (fig. 6.1), Kjetland has determined that prior schistosomiasis occurred in 22% of 1,057 girls between the ages of 10 and 12 and was linked to their genital symptoms [35]. Today FGS is one of KwaZulu-Natal's important gynecologic conditions. FGS and consequently HIV/AIDS might be prevented if KwaZulu-Natal's girls received regular praziquantel treatment, especially if MDA was started at a young age in order to prevent the onset of genital lesions. Indeed, an economic modeling group based at Yale University and led by Dr. Alison Galvani working with Dr. Martial Ndeffo Mbah used data from Zimbabwe to

Figure 6.1.
Map of the Ugu district in South Africa. From [35].

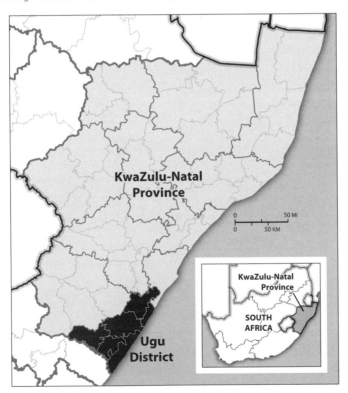

determine that preventing schistosomiasis through MDA with praziquantel is one of the most cost-effective means to prevent HIV/AIDS [36].

Based on such studies, I believe there is an urgent need to scale-up mass distribution and MDA for praziquantel in KwaZulu-Natal, where only a tiny percentage of the population currently receives treatment. Presumably, children would need to receive MDA beginning at a young age in order to prevent the onset of genital lesions. According to some investigators, once the ulcerative lesions start to appear on the cervix, uterus, and lower genital tract, a conduit for the HIV virus has already been established, so receiving praziquantel later in life would not be nearly as beneficial. Given findings that Tanzania also has an important *S. haematobium* schistosomiasis–HIV/AIDS link, it is worth exploring how MDA with praziquantel could be boosted there. Indeed, there is a need to greatly expand praziquantel MDA throughout sub-Saharan Africa. My friend and colleague Professor Alan Fenwick at the Imperial College London–based SCI (Schistosomiasis Control Initiative) is working hard toward that goal.

In South Africa and elsewhere in sub-Saharan Africa, female genital schistosomiasis represents one of the most important yet ignored cofactors promoting the HIV/AIDS epidemic.

As an alternative technology, my group at the Sabin Vaccine Institute and Texas Children's Hospital Center for Vaccine Development is also developing a schistosomiasis vaccine that might also one day become an important backdoor AIDS prevention technology [37, 38]. The schistosomiasis vaccine is currently undergoing phase 1 clinical testing for safety and immunogenicity in Houston, with hopes that clinical trials will commence in sub-Saharan Africa.

In 2014, the *New York Times* ran a front-page story on the public health threat to Africa's girls and women posed by FGS [39]. Titled "A Simple Theory, and a Proposal, on HIV in Africa," the piece has so far generated only modest international attention and resources. Despite overwhelming evidence pointing to the links between FGS and HIV/AIDS, programs of schistosomiasis control and prevention have yet to be embraced by the global AIDS public health community or major treatment and prevention programs such as PEPFAR and GFATM. I have been working with the US Congress to better integrate NTD MDA into these programs for HIV/AIDS, and we are beginning to gain some traction and to spur interest and global action.

Moreover, South Africa itself has an important biomedical research structure, among the most sophisticated on the African continent. The major pieces include an important South African Medical Research Council, and a Wellcome Trust Africa Centre in KwaZulu-Natal, among others. Its universities are the only ones that compete internationally in QS rankings [29]. These institutions have unparalleled opportunities to investigate schistosomiasis and HIV/AIDS coinfections, as well as how NTDs interface with other big three diseases and NCDs.

Concluding Remarks

Africa's two leading economies are simultaneously major contributors to the continent's disease burden from NTDs, in addition to HIV/AIDS and malaria. All three disease categories are linked and would benefit from greater government commitment, especially for NTDs. Nigeria in particular is the single largest contributor to NTDs in Africa, including intestinal helminth infections, schistosomiasis, LF, and onchocerciasis, while South Africa is home to a horrific but almost ignored problem with female genital schistosomiasis, a major cofactor in its HIV/AIDS epidemic. It is essential that both nations scale up MDA efforts, and both are severely underachieving in this aspect, especially given their recent economic growth. Both countries require internal champions to expand MDA for NTDs and to advocate with parliamentarians and cabinet ministers. Simultaneously, both Nigeria and South Africa have enormous potential to contribute to research and development in the fight against NTDs. Their major research institutes and universities represent untapped sources of innovation.

Summary Points

1. In 2015, WHO determined that 35% of the eligible population in its African region is receiving access to essential NTD medicines. In all, 229.5 million people received MDA in 2013. During the same period, the World Bank estimates that Africa's economy has grown by an average of 4.4% annually. Quite possibly the two are linked.
2. By far, Nigeria and South Africa represent the largest economies in sub-Saharan Africa, yet these two nations also suffer from widespread NTDs.

3. Nigeria: With a GDP of more than $0.5 trillion, Nigeria boasts the largest economy in sub-Saharan Africa.

   a. However, despite this massive growth, widespread poverty is rampant—almost 150 million Nigerians have virtually no income.

   b. Nigeria is also "ground zero" for the world's high-prevalence NTDs. Nigeria ranks first among African nations in almost every high-prevalence NTD disease category, and it ranks first globally in cases of schistosomiasis and onchocerciasis and third globally for LF.

   c. Until recently, Nigeria has not exercised the political will necessary to provide MDA for its population's NTDs, but the government has recently launched a "master plan" for these diseases, working in collaboration with several American and European nongovernmental organizations.

4. South Africa: NTDs are also widespread in Africa's only G20 nation, especially in KwaZulu-Natal.

   a. Schistosomiasis is one of South Africa's highest-prevalence NTDs, and FGS is devastating South Africa's girls and women, representing a major cofactor in its HIV/AIDS epidemic, especially in KwaZulu-Natal.

   b. There is an urgent need to expand MDA coverage for schistosomiasis in South Africa, which also represents a highly cost-effective means to prevent HIV/AIDS. So far, large-scale AIDS treatment and prevention programs have not embraced MDA for NTDs such as schistosomiasis, but it is hoped that this will begin to change soon.

5. Africa's two leading economies are simultaneously major contributors to the continent's disease burden from NTDs, in addition to HIV/AIDS and malaria.

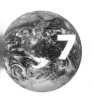

Saudi Arabia and Neighboring Conflict Zones of the Middle East and North African Region

Until relatively recently, the region known as MENA—Middle East and North Africa—was not considered a major "hot zone" for NTDs. However, emerging information indicates that MENA is an important area for the world's neglected diseases, especially NTDs that are now arising in ISIS-occupied conflict areas in Syria, Iraq, and Libya, as well as in Yemen.

Kingdom of Saudi Arabia

Despite the fact that it is a wealthy G20 nation, Saudi Arabia has an extreme vulnerability to the NTDs. These diseases threaten the health and economy of the country for multiple reasons. First, even though the kingdom has vast oil wealth and GDP that will soon reach $1 trillion, a segment of Saudi Arabian society lives in poverty. Much of the nation's poverty and its impoverished population is hidden and not easily viewed. According to a 2013 article in the *Guardian*, of Saudi Arabia's population of almost 30 million, approximately 2–4 million of the native Saudis live below the nation's poverty line (estimated then at $530 per month), despite government efforts to aggressively invest internally as a means to address this problem [1]. Indeed, during drives with the American Embassy staff in my role as US science envoy, it was possible to see firsthand evidence of acute poverty in the kingdom, but it was seldom obvious and required traveling away from major thoroughfares to find it.

NTDs are strongly associated with Saudi Arabia's poverty, along with factors related to climate. As of 2013, schistosomiasis was still endemic in Al-Bahah Province in the southwestern part of the country [2]. Cutaneous leishmaniasis is also widespread and was epidemic in the Al-Hassa oasis during the 1980s; both *Leishmania tropica* and *L. major* are present, although a national control program focused on case detection, vector control, and other measures is reducing the total number of cases [3]. Whether recent drops in oil prices will expand poverty and poverty-related diseases in Saudi Arabia remains to be seen.

A second driving force for NTDs in Saudi Arabia is its geographic location, sandwiched between two major conflict zones: ISIS-held Syria and Iraq to the north and Yemen to the south. The risk of NTDs from ISIS areas is discussed below, but even in the years prior to the Syrian conflict, Yemen was also "ground zero" for NTDs in the MENA region, with some of the highest prevalence rates of schistosomiasis, fascioliasis, intestinal helminth infections, and trachoma, among others [4].

The major driving forces that promote NTDs in the Kingdom of Saudi Arabia include hidden poverty, geographic proximity to conflict zones, and the annual pilgrimage.

Superimposed on these two socioeconomic forces—poverty and conflict—is the Hajj, the annual Muslim pilgrimage to Mecca, which brings 2–3 million visitors to Saudi Arabia during the last month of the Islamic calendar. The majority of the pilgrims arrive from Muslim countries belonging to the Organisation of Islamic Cooperation (OIC), which includes MENA countries, many sub-Saharan African nations, and large Islamic Asian countries such as Bangladesh and Indonesia. Previously, I found that OIC countries (fig. 7.1) are also disproportionately affected by poverty and NTDs, especially intestinal helminth infections, schistosomiasis, trachoma, and leprosy [5]. From an epidemiological framework, the Hajj is a vast mixing bowl that has the potential to spread NTDs and other emerging infections across the Muslim world. There are particular concerns about respiratory viruses such as avian influenza and MERS coronavirus, but it is also believed that during the 1990s the Hajj may have introduced dengue fever into Jeddah, the location of the major international airport closest to Mecca. Nucleic acid sequencing of Saudi Arabian dengue virus strains suggests that it could have been first introduced by African pilgrims infected with an Asian genotype [6]. The number of dengue cases has been reported on the rise in the years between 2006 and 2013, and some investi-

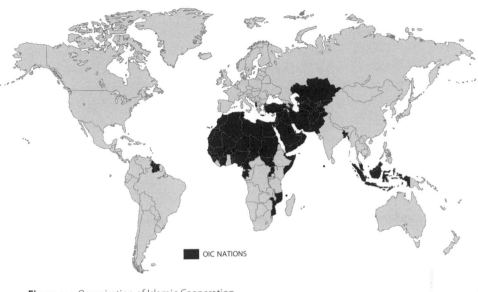

Figure 7.1. Organisation of Islamic Cooperation
(OIC) nations. From [5].

gators have called for stepped-up control measures to combat dengue and
related vector-borne virus infections [7].

Still another major issue related to NTDs in Saudi Arabia is their possible links with noncommunicable diseases. NCDs are on a steep rise throughout the Arab world [8]. During my time in Saudi Arabia, I was impressed by
high NCD rates among its population, especially type 2 diabetes, which
leads to high rates of complications and has now become a major public
health threat to the nation [9, 10]. In the near future, it will become crucial
to better understand how some of the emerging NTDs such as dengue fever
or MERS coronavirus infection interface with diabetes and
other NCDs in Saudi Arabia. For example, as I discussed
earlier about India, diabetes and hypertension were shown
to be important comorbidities with dengue fever [11].

Although the MENA region, and the Kingdom of Saudi
Arabia in particular, is at great risk for both emerging NTDs
and NCDs, as well as comorbidities from these two major
groups of diseases, I am also impressed with overall level
of Saudi innovation and their capacity to one day develop new control tools,
including new drugs, diagnostics, and vaccines. Today, the top universities

*NCDs with NTD
coinfections will
become an important
health concern for
Saudi Arabia in the
coming years.*

Increasingly, Saudi Arabia will need to step-up its ability to develop and test innovative strategies to counter its emerging NTDs.

in the MENA region are based in Saudi Arabia [12], and during my visits as US science envoy, I have admired their commitment to translational research and development, that is, the translation of basic scientific discoveries from the laboratory bench to the clinic. Indeed, the future will require new technologies to combat the diseases emerging from ISIS-held territories and Yemen. Since many of those diseases are of regional importance (rather than ones having a global impact), they are unlikely to be targeted by major multinational pharmaceutical companies. Saudi-led innovation may become a critical factor in fighting the new NTDs arising out of conflict in the Middle East.

Beyond Saudi Arabia: Poverty and NTDs in the MENA region

The situation of poverty amidst wealth is not unique to Saudi Arabia in the MENA region. The 21 major countries of the MENA region include Algeria, Bahrain, Djibouti, Egypt, Iran, Iraq, Israel, Jordan, Kuwait, Lebanon, Libya, Malta, Morocco, Oman, the Palestinian territories, Qatar, Saudi Arabia, Syria, Tunisia, United Arab Emirates, and Yemen. As shown in table 7.1, almost 400 million people live in the MENA nations, including 17%, or approximately 65 million people, who live on less than $2 per day [4]. In my analysis conducted prior to the Syrian civil war, Yemen had the highest concentration of poverty (47% living on less than $2 per day), while Egypt had the largest number of impoverished people [4].

According to the World Bank, the economic development of the MENA region is currently imperiled because of the destroyed economies in ISIS-occupied countries, the pressure created by refugees in neighboring Jordan and Lebanon, and the post–Arab Spring transitions, accompanied by ongoing destabilizing dynamics in Egypt and Tunisia. Prolonged and protracted wars and political instability are projected to ensure continued sluggish economic growth and high unemployment, while low oil prices are adversely affecting the Arabian Gulf monarchies [13]. One of the few possible economic improvements will likely occur in Iran, with the lifting of sanctions following the 2015 nuclear agreements.

Table 7.1. Population of the countries of the MENA region and percentage living in poverty

Country	Total population	% of the population living on less than US$2 per day
Algeria	36.0 million	24
Bahrain	1.3 million	
Djibouti	0.9 million	
Egypt	80.4 million	18
Iran	75.1 million	8
Iraq	31.5 million	6
Israel	7.6 million	
Jordan	6.5 million	4
Kuwait	3.1 million	
Lebanon	4.3 million	
Libya	6.6 million	
Malta	0.4 million	
Morocco	31.9 million	14
Oman	3.1 million	
Palestinian territories	4.1 million	
Qatar	1.7 million	
Saudi Arabia	29.2 million	
Syria	22.5 million	
Tunisia	10.5 million	13
United Arab Emirates	5.4 million	
Yemen	23.6 million	47
TOTAL MENA	392 million	16.9

Source: [4], doi:10.1371/journal.pntd.0001475.t001.
Note: Data for poverty in Iraq from [5]. When no number appears, it indicates that the data are not available.

NTDs are flourishing in this setting of economic stress. Shown in table 7.2 is my 2012 ranking of the NTDs affecting most of the 65 million people living in extreme poverty in the MENA region, led by the intestinal helminth infections, schistosomiasis, a foodborne trematode infection known as fascioliasis, and two forms of cutaneous leishmaniasis caused by *L. tropica* and *L. major*, respectively. When these diseases are broken down by country, as shown in table 7.3, the two nations with the highest concentration of pov-

Table 7.2. Ranking of NTDs in the MENA region by prevalence

Disease	Estimated or reported number of cases	% of global burden of disease
Ascariasis	22.3 million	3
Schistosomiasis	12.7 million	6
Trichuriasis	9.0 million	1
Hookworm infection	4.7 million	1
Fascioliasis	0.9 million	36
Trachoma	0.6 million	1
Anthroponotic cutaneous leishmaniasis (*L. tropica*)	0.04 million	Not determined
Zoonotic cutaneous leishmaniasis (*L. major*)	0.03 million	Not determined
Leprosy	<0.01 million	3
Rift Valley fever	>1,000 cases during outbreaks	Not determined
Brucellosis	Not determined	Not determined
Dengue	Not determined	Not determined
Echinococcosis	Not determined	Not determined
Crimean-Congo hemorrhagic fever	Not determined	Not determined
Alkhurma hemorrhagic fever	Not determined	Not determined
Toxoplasmosis	Not determined	Not determined
Visceral leishmaniasis	Not determined	Not determined

Source: [4], doi:10.1371/journal.pntd.0001475.t002.

erty in the years before the takeovers by ISIS—Egypt and Yemen—also represented the leading countries where most of the NTDs are widespread. An exception is the prevalence and incident rates of cutaneous leishmaniasis in Syria, Iraq, and Saudi Arabia. Morocco also had a surprising burden of NTDs [4].

The major neglected parasitic diseases in the MENA region include intestinal helminth infections, leishmaniasis, and malaria. LF still occurs in Egypt.

These numbers were updated in 2015 (table 7.4), revealing that intestinal helminth infections remain widespread in the MENA region, as does schistosomiasis, especially in Yemen [12]. As in India, dengue fever has emerged in Egypt, Oman, Saudi Arabia, Syria, and Yemen, where approximately two million new or "incident" cases occurred in 2013 and presumably are continuing annually [12, 14].

Table 7.3. MENA countries with the highest prevalence of NTDs

Disease	Estimated or reported number of cases	Country with highest prevalence (no. of cases)	Country with second-highest prevalence (no. of cases)	Country with third-highest prevalence (no. of cases)	Country with fourth-highest prevalence (no. of cases)
Ascariasis	22.3 million	Egypt (8.3 million)	Yemen (5.8 million)	Iran (5.1 million)	Morocco (1.3. million)
Schistosomiasis	12.7 million	Egypt (7.2 million)	Yemen (2.9 million)	Algeria (2.3 million)	Libya (0.3 million)
Trichuriasis	9.0 million	Morocco (3.2 million)	Egypt (1.7 million)	Iran (1.6 million)	Yemen (1.5 million)
Hookworm infection	4.7 million	Egypt (3.6 million)	Iran (0.4 million)	Saudi Arabia (0.4 million)	Oman (0.2 million)
Fascioliasis	0.9 million	Egypt (830,000)	Yemen (37,000)	Iran (10,000)	Not determined
Trachoma	0.6 million	Yemen (204,984)	Algeria (143,356)	Iraq (140,697)	Libya (24,244)
Anthroponotic cutaneous leishmaniasis (*L. tropica*)	0.04 million	Syria (27,739)	Iran (8,649)	Morocco (1,697)	Yemen (179)
Zoonotic cutaneous leishmaniasis (*L. major*)	0.03 million	Iran (18,175)	Saudi Arabia (4,238)	Morocco (3,431)	Tunisia (2,750)
Leprosy	<0.01 million	Egypt (912)	Yemen (424)	Iran (81)	Morocco (72)

Source: [4], doi:10.1371/journal.pntd.0001475.t003.

Table 7.4. Revised estimates of NTDs in MENA

Disease	Number of cases	Comments
Ascariasis	24.3 million	Total infected population
Schistosomiasis	9.2 million	Population requiring preventive chemotherapy for schistosomiasis annually in WHO eastern Mediterranean region, 2013, minus Somalia and Sudan (which are not ordinarily considered MENA countries)
Trichuriasis	8.7 million	Total infected population
Hookworm infection	4.6 million	Total infected population
Dengue	2.0 million	Total "apparent" cases in Egypt, Oman, Saudi Arabia, Syria, and Yemen
Lymphatic filariasis (LF)	550,172	Population requiring preventive chemotherapy for LF in WHO eastern Mediterranean region, 2013, minus Somalia and Sudan (which are not ordinarily considered MENA countries)
Cutaneous leishmaniasis	465,700 to 810,000	Total incidence of the combined regions designated as Mediterranean and Middle East to central Asia
Malaria	107,267	Total confirmed cases in 2013 in WHO eastern Mediterranean region endemic countries reporting: Algeria, Iran, Saudi Arabia, Yemen
Visceral leishmaniasis	6,200 to 12,000	Total incidence of the combined regions designated as Mediterranean and Middle East to central Asia
MERS	>1,000	Laboratory-confirmed cases
Leprosy	<1,000	Registered cases in WHO eastern Mediterranean region 2013 minus Pakistan, Somalia, and Sudan
Trachoma	Endemic	Reported as "endemic" in Egypt, Iraq, Libya, Yemen

Source: [12], doi:10.1371/journal.pntd.0003852.

Cutaneous leishmaniasis remains widespread, as does malaria and trachoma in selected countries [12].

Conflict and New Catastrophic NTDs

The 2014 Ebola outbreak in West Africa reminded us about the links between conflict or postconflict and the emergence of an NTD. As was pointed out by Tulane University's Dan Bausch and Lara Schwarz at McGill University, and others, Ebola rapidly spread in Guinea, Liberia, and Sierra Leone in 2014 not so much because these countries are in the tropics—although that might represent a part of the answer—but instead mostly because these nations had only recently emerged from armed conflict that had spawned horrific atrocities. As a result, the three most affected West African countries had previously experienced massive breakdowns in basic infrastructure, especially health systems, in addition to deforestation, human migrations, and collapsed economies [15]. Thus it was potent social forces that helped to propel the 2014 Ebola virus epidemic, and although we designate them as neglected *tropical* diseases, the NTDs are first and foremost diseases of poverty—but also diseases arising out poverty in conjunction with conflict.

The Ebola virus outbreak of 2014–15 exposed the links between conflict, postconflict, and the emergence of a catastrophic infection. In some ways Ebola represents "version 3.0" of a trend we have been seeing all too regularly since the end of the twentieth century.

During my TV and radio interviews at the height of the Ebola epidemic in the summer of 2014, I often pointed out that such links between war and outbreaks of epidemic NTDs were nothing new. During World War II, louseborne typhus decimated populations in Europe; while during the last 25 years of the twentieth century, human African trypanosomiasis (sleeping sickness) caused hundreds of thousands of deaths in Angola, Democratic Republic of Congo, and Sudan following decades of civil unrest; and throughout the 1980s and '90s, kala-azar killed more than 100,000 people fleeing conflicts in southern Sudan [16]. In this sense, Ebola was "version 3.0" of a link between NTDs and African conflict that began during the 1970s.

ISIS-Occupied Conflict Zones and NTDs

In my newest role as US science envoy, I have been emphasizing that version 4.0 of the NTD-conflict interface might likely be the diseases resulting from the atrocities and civil war in ISIS (Islamic State of Iraq and Syria)-held areas of Syria, Iraq, and Libya, as well as in Yemen [12, 16]. ISIS holds vast territories in these countries but has shown little if any interest in preserving any semblance of public health infrastructure. Although it has been difficult for WHO or other international health agencies to gain access to the conflict zones in the MENA region, it has been possible to glimpse the diseases arising in these battlegrounds from refugees spilling across the borders into Egypt, Jordan, Lebanon, and Turkey. For instance, we have seen the reemergence of polio and measles in these areas, because vaccination programs have been halted or interrupted. Today, measles remains one of the great killers of young children, resulting in close to 100,000 deaths annually worldwide [17]. We may also be witnessing the reversal of previous successes in the campaign against polio, just as we were on the verge of eradicating it in the MENA region.

The next big wave in the NTD-conflict interaction will be diseases arising out of ISIS-occupied conflict zones in the Middle East and North Africa (MENA).

In addition to the major childhood diseases, NTDs have also emerged or reemerged. One particularly troublesome disease arising from the conflict in Syria is a cutaneous form of leishmaniasis, which is quite different from kala-azar (visceral leishmaniasis). Cutaneous leishmaniasis has affected the Middle East for centuries, where it has a variety of names, including "Baghdad boil" or "Aleppo evil" [18]. It is also sometimes known as "one year sore," referring to the time it takes for the characteristic ulcerative lesion to heal. In Syria and nearby regions, a major cause of Aleppo evil is the protozoan parasite *Leishmania tropica*, which is transmitted by *Phlebotomus* sandflies. *L. tropica* can cause a permanent scar, and when this happens on

Figure 7.2.
Left: Syrian boy with probable leishmaniasis lesions on his face waits for intralesional injections of an antiparasitic drug. *Right:* Piled-up garbage in Aleppo offers new habitats for *Phlebotomus* sandfly proliferation. Photos by Hannah Lucinda Smith.

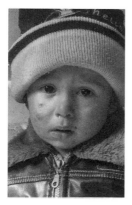
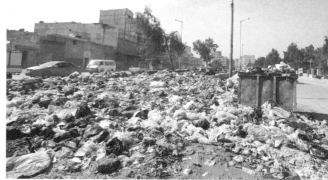

the face, it can be highly disfiguring and socially stigmatizing, especially for young girls and women. To reduce the likelihood of permanent scarring, the lesions on the face are treated by injecting them with a chemical antiparasitic agent that contains antimony (fig. 7.2).

The problem in Syria, however, is that with the breakdowns in health infrastructure in Aleppo and elsewhere, the treatments are often not available. Compounding the problem is that with the collapse of city services in Aleppo or other urban centers, refuse has piled up, which creates great habitats for *Phlebotomus* sandflies and encourages their proliferation. In addition to severe problems with sanitation and waste disposal, there has been an overall collapse in the public health system [3]. As a result, transmission of leishmaniasis is now widespread and in some cases out of control in Syria and neighboring areas.

The major NTDs arising out of conflict zones in MENA include leishmaniasis, MERS coronavirus infection, and brucellosis, among others.

In 2014, a group at the Al-Imam Mohammed Ibn Saud Islamic University in Riyadh, Saudi Arabia, chronicled their findings and published a report in *PLOS NTDs* showing a dramatic surge in the number of cases of cutaneous leishmaniasis in Syria (fig. 7.3) [3]. In 2012, more than 50,000 cases occurred, and there is no

Figure 7.3.
Cases of cutaneous leishmaniasis reported in the Middle East, 1989–2011. From [3].

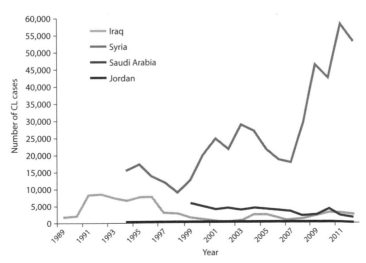

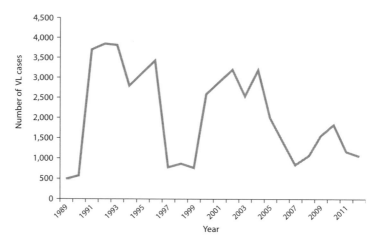

Figure 7.4.
Cases of kala-azar (visceral leishmaniasis, VL)
reported in Iraq, 1989–2011. From [3].

evidence that this number has since declined. Similarly in Iraq, there were
two major peaks of kala-azar (visceral leishmaniasis, VL) over the past two
decades that roughly correspond to Iraqi conflicts, including the first Gulf
War (Operation Desert Storm) in 1990–91 and the Iraq War (Operation Iraqi
Freedom) more than 10 years later (fig. 7.4) [3].

Emerging Virus Infections

Additional NTDs now appearing because of MENA conflicts are those that
arise from open borders and the trafficking of animals, which leads to zoonotic diseases. Such zoonotic NTDs include the Middle Eastern Respiratory
Syndrome (MERS) coronavirus that emerged following transmission from
camels to humans on the Arabian Peninsula in 2012, and brucellosis [12].

The situation with MERS coronavirus is of particular concern because
of its potential to create epidemics across war-torn areas of the MENA region. The first known human MERS infections occurred in 2012, ultimately
resulting in more than 1,000 cases and 400 deaths by the spring of 2015 [19,
20]. MERS produces a severe and devastating lung infection that can lead to
respiratory failure. The disease is especially lethal among the elderly and

those with underlying NCDs. Most of these cases in the MENA region have occurred in Saudi Arabia (1,010), followed by the United Arab Emirates (76), Jordan (19), and Qatar (13) [20].

MERS coronavirus represents an important emerging threat to the MENA region.

The MERS coronavirus is believed to be widespread among dromedary camels on the Arabian Peninsula and possibly elsewhere in the MENA region. Many of the human cases have resulted from contact with camels or camel-derived products. However, human-to-human transmission has occurred among household contacts and in hospital settings [19]. Hospital-acquired MERS is also the basis of the large South Korean outbreak that occurred in 2015. So far, human-to-human transmission has not been sustained in the MENA region, but an important question is whether this situation might change because of the combination of crowding and large movements of human populations in ISIS-occupied areas or refugee camps.

The MERS coronavirus is not the only new virus to surface in the MENA region. Others with the potential for epidemic spread include two viral infections transmitted by ticks: Crimean-Congo hemorrhagic fever and Alkhurma hemorrhagic fever [4]. The former caused an outbreak in Iran in 2008, while one also occurred in Oman; the latter is a flaviviral infection (as is the dengue virus) that, like MERS, emerged on the Arabian Peninsula. Beginning in the 1990s, dengue fever reemerged in Jeddah and elsewhere in western Saudi Arabia, and outbreaks have since appeared in both Saudi Arabia and Yemen. A large number of dengue fever cases now also occur in Egypt, possibly linked to health infrastructure breakdowns associated with the political instability there following the Arab Spring. It is reasonable to believe that dengue could

Dengue and Rift Valley fevers represent important arboviral threats to the MENA region.

become as widespread in MENA as it is in India or Indonesia today. Rift Valley fever is another mosquito-borne virus that emerged in 2000 in southwestern Saudi Arabia and across the border in Yemen [4].

Summary Points

1. The Kingdom of Saudi Arabia is a wealthy G20 economy, yet it is highly vulnerable to NTDs.

    a. A major factor is a (mostly) hidden burden of poverty, with 2–4 million Saudi citizens living below the poverty level. Schistosomiasis and leishmaniasis represent important endemic NTDs.

    b. A second socioeconomic force is war and conflict, and the resulting diseases emerging out of the ISIS-held areas to the north and Yemen to the south.

    c. A third factor is the annual Hajj and the huge influx of pilgrims from OIC countries where NTDs are endemic. The Hajj may explain how dengue fever perhaps first emerged in Jeddah during the 1990s.

    d. NCDs, including type 2 diabetes, are simultaneously on the rise in Saudi Arabia, and NTD and NCD comorbidities may represent an important disease paradigm in the kingdom in the coming years.

    e. Such disease pressures will demand a new level of innovation from Saudi Arabia's major universities and research institutes, with a focus on translational medicine research and development.

2. Even beyond Middle Eastern conflicts, poverty is widespread in many parts of the MENA region. An estimated 65 million out of almost 400 million people live on less than $2 per day.

3. The major NTDs found in impoverished areas of the MENA region include helminth infections (e.g., intestinal helminth infections and schistosomiasis) and vector-borne diseases (e.g., cutaneous leishmaniasis, malaria, and dengue).

4. A new generation of NTDs and other infectious diseases is emerging from the atrocities and civil wars in ISIS-held areas of Syria, Iraq, and Libya, as well as in Yemen.

5. The diseases arising out of conflict zones include reemerging polio and measles, as well as selected NTDs, such as cutaneous leishmaniasis ("Aleppo evil").

6. The emerging viral NTDs are cause for great concern. MERS coronavirus appeared in 2012, with more than 1,000 reported cases on the Arabian Peninsula. Dengue fever is now an important NTD in Saudi Arabia, Egypt, and elsewhere.

8 The Americas

Argentina, Brazil, and Mexico

Latin American countries exhibit some of the highest GINI indices in the world today. Developed by Corrado Gini, an Italian academic working in the early decades of the twentieth century, his index (or coefficient, which divides the index by 100) measures national inequalities. At one end, a GINI index of zero indicates that income levels are evenly distributed such that everyone has the same income, while a GINI index of 100 means that one person holds all of the money and resources. In recent years, globally, South Africa traditionally has had the highest recorded GINI index of any single country—65.0 (GINI coefficient of 0.65) in 2011, according to the World Bank [1]. Some fragile and oil-rich African nations such as Equatorial Guinea may exceed even this level.

Overall, however, Latin American countries have maintained the highest GINI indices. Spending time in any major Latin American city such as São Paulo or Rio de Janeiro in Brazil or in Mexico City, Tegucigalpa, Panama City, Guatemala City, makes it clear why. The differences between the "haves" and the "have-nots" are astounding. I do a fair bit of work in Latin America, especially Brazil, where we have been codeveloping our human hookworm and schistosomiasis vaccines. The economic differences are often jarring. For example, in Rio de Janeiro there are luxury hotels on Copacabana and Ipanema Beaches, and just a few miles away near FIOCRUZ (Fundação Oswaldo Cruz, the location of our scientific collaborators who work to develop new innovations for NTDs) are the *favelas* where devastating poverty rules the day. In Tegucigalpa or in Guatemala City, the wealthy are typically separated from the poor and live behind tall and impenetrable fences topped by barbed wire. This trend of high GINI indices now extends beyond Latin America into Texas. For instance, my city of Houston's GINI index also exceeds 50, as do several other Texas cities [2].

According to the *Economist*, Latin America's income inequality increased steadily from 1980 to 2000 [3]. Overall, the region's GINI coefficient remains incredibly high, at around 0.50, one of the highest for any major global or World Bank region. Such high GINI coefficients have not slowed Latin America's economy. During the first decade of the 2000s its economic growth was impressive, averaging 5% annually between the years 2003 and 2012 [4]. It has since slowed to only 2.0–2.5% of its GDP [4]. However, that previous decade of economic growth helped to lift an estimated 70 million people in the region out of extreme poverty and allowed Latin America's middle class to expand by an estimated 50% [4].

Just as in the rest of the "blue marble," such robust economic growth in Latin America has left behind the region's most impoverished people. Also according to the World Bank, of the more than 600 million people who live in the Latin American and Caribbean (LAC) region, 130 million remain "chronically poor" [4]. I have previously reported that approximately 50 million people in the LAC region live below the 2005–14 World Bank poverty figure of $1.25 per day, while 100 million live on less than $2 per day [5].

NTDs are pervasive among the LAC region's "bottom 100 million" [5]. Shown in table 8.1 is a ranking of the leading NTDs by prevalence [6–9], led by the three major intestinal helminth infections and schistosomiasis, in

Table 8.1. The leading NTDs of the LAC region's "bottom 100 million"

NTD	Number of people infected in LAC (in millions)	Reference
Ascariasis	86.0	[6]
Trichuriasis	72.2	[6]
Hookworm infection	30.3	[6]
Chagas disease	5.7	[7]
Schistosomiasis	1.5	[8]
Malaria	0.4 (confirmed cases); 25 million people at high risk	[9]

addition to more than five million people living with Chagas disease, according to WHO. Chagas disease (American trypanosomiasis caused by *Trypanosoma cruzi*) is a serious and debilitating heart infection transmitted by triatomine kissing bugs, as well as mother-to-child transmission. It is almost exclusively a disease of extreme poverty linked to poor-quality housing where kissing bugs thrive, among other low socioeconomic and ecologic factors. The vast majority of cases are found in Latin America. Moreover, there are approximately 25 million people at high risk for malaria in the Americas, mostly from the nonfatal but debilitating form caused by *Plasmodium vivax* [9]. Three countries—Brazil, Colombia, and Venezuela—account for almost three-quarters of the LAC regions malaria cases [9].

Today, the three wealthiest G20 countries in the LAC region are Argentina, Brazil, and Mexico. With a combined population of 377 million people [10], these three nations account for just over one-half of LAC's population. However, with a combined GDP of just under $4.2 trillion [10], Argentina, Brazil, and Mexico simultaneously represent three-quarters of Latin America's economy (box 8.1). Despite such vast wealth, Latin America's three wealthiest economies simultaneously account for most of the region's extreme poverty and NTDs, including most of the schistosomiasis and Chagas disease, and almost one-half the intestinal helminth infections and malaria.

Brazil alone accounts for 42% of LAC's malaria cases [9] and, according to WHO, 95% of the region's schistosomiasis burden [8]. WHO also finds that together Argentina, Brazil, and Mexico are responsible for almost one-half of LAC's children requiring regular deworming for intestinal

Latin America and its three wealthiest countries— Argentina, Brazil, and Mexico—are representative of the "classic" blue marble health paradox: most of Latin America's people suffering from NTDs live in the region's wealthiest countries.

Box 8.1.
Argentina, Brazil, Mexico
75% of the region's economy (GDP)
95% of the region's schistosomiasis
61% of the region's Chagas disease
48% of the region's intestinal helminth infections
42% of the region's malaria

helminth infections [11], and 61% of people in Latin America living with Chagas disease [7]. Therefore, Argentina, Brazil, and Mexico present the "classic" blue marble health paradox—most of the region's people infected with NTDs are living in its wealthiest countries.

Argentina

Argentina has a population of just over 40 million people and the LAC's third-largest economy, with a GDP exceeding $0.5 trillion [12]. At the turn of the twenty-first century, its economy collapsed and Argentina defaulted on its debt, but since then the nation has rebounded, recovering through steady economic growth. By some metrics, according to the Nobel laureate economist Paul Krugman, the Argentine economy has surpassed that of Brazil [13].

Argentine economic growth, however, has also succeeded in creating two major national divides: rural versus urban and north versus south. Argentina's north, including (1) the northwestern part of the country centered in the province of Salta, (2) the northern Gran Chaco region, and (3) the northeastern Mesopotamian region, suffers from high rates of poverty and disease. The Gran Chaco, home to almost 10 million people, is a large, hot, lowland region that begins in northern Argentina and extends into Bolivia, Paraguay, and even parts of Brazil (fig. 8.1). In a paper in *PLOS NTDs* I previously identified the Gran Chaco as one of 10 major global "hotspots" for NTDs, because of its high disease burden from intestinal helminth infections and Chagas disease, among other NTDs [14].

According to Drs. Gonzalo M. Vazquez-Prokopec, Ricardo E. Gürtler, and their colleagues at the University of Buenos Aires, the Gran Chaco is well suited to promote Chagas disease and other NTDs because of a "perfect storm" of factors, including poverty, rural populations of low densities, a subsistence economy, and weak health systems. They estimate, for instance, that the prevalence of Chagas disease in the Gran Chaco may range as high as 45%. Moreover, there is evidence for emerging insecticide resistance that has thwarted efforts to eliminate the triatomine Chagas disease vector, *Triatoma infestans*, whereas similar efforts have been successful elsewhere in Latin America's other Southern Cone countries [15]. Overall, Gürtler and

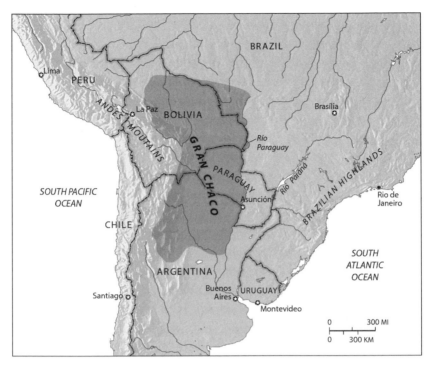

Figure 8.1.
Approximate location of the Gran Chaco region in northern
Argentina, Bolivia, Brazil, and Paraguay. From https://en.wikipedia
.org/wiki/Gran_Chaco.

his colleagues have found that triatomines in the Gran Chaco exhibit complicated ecological patterns that must also be taken into consideration when embarking on elimination efforts that emphasize vector control [16].

Today, the world's largest numbers of people living with Chagas disease (1.5 million according to WHO) now live in Argentina [7], with the overwhelming majority in northern part of the country. Moreover, intestinal helminth infections are also widespread, including an unusual type found in northern Argentina known as strongyloidiasis. *Strongyloides stercoralis*, the causative agent of this disease, has the unusual feature of being one of the only intestinal helminths to have the ability to replicate in the human body and cause a severe hyperinfection syndrome associated with a high mortality rate. An important nongovernmental organization based in Bue-

Northern Argentina, especially its Gran Chaco region, is a global hotspot for NTDs, especially for intestinal helminth infections and Chagas disease.

nos Aires known as (Fundación) Mundo Sano (Healthy World) is working to reduce the disease burden from Chagas disease, intestinal helminth infections, and other NTDs in northern Argentina [17].

Mundo Sano aggressively works to expand access to diagnosis and treatment for Chagas disease in northern Argentina. Headed by Dr. Silvia Gold, the organization is particularly committed to treating *T. cruzi*–infected patients with the drug benznidazole, which, if used early enough in the course of the illness, can cure patients and prevent the onset of severe heart disease. Mundo Sano also facilitated the local manufacture of benznidazole in order to make it even more accessible. Sadly, less than 1% of people living with Chagas disease in Latin America are diagnosed and treated for their disease. In addition, Mundo Sano has created mass treatment programs for intestinal helminth infections in northern Argentina, which includes the diagnosis and treatment of patients with strongyloidiasis [17].

Brazil

Brazil has the largest population (more than 200 million people) and the largest economy (a GDP that exceeds $2 trillion) in Latin America and the LAC region [18]. It also has a significant burden of poverty and the highest NTD disease burden in the Americas. Over the course of a decade beginning in 2003, Brazil's economy grew steadily, and millions of the poorest people in the country were lifted out of extreme poverty [18]. There was even a 6% drop in Brazil's GINI index. However, by 2012, the nation's GINI index remained at 52.7, one of the highest of any large nation [1]. Moreover, in recent years the Brazilian economy has slowed considerably, in part owing to a massive corruption and bribery scandal involving Brazil's publicly owned oil producer, Petrobras [19]. The end result is that the expansion of Brazil's economy during the past decade is over for now, and ultimately left behind are approximately 6.8% of its population, more than 13 million people, living in extreme poverty on less than $2 per day [20]. Similar to Argentina, Brazil's extreme poverty is not evenly distributed, with much of it is currently centered in northeastern states—where up to 25% of the pop-

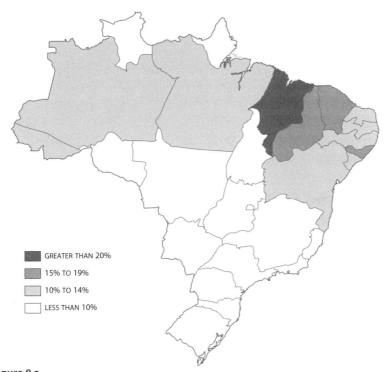

Figure 8.2.
Poverty map of Brazil, 2010, showing the percentage of the
population living in extreme poverty (less than US$70 per
month). From [21].

ulation lives in extreme poverty—as well as in the Amazon region, where
many indigenous peoples live (fig. 8.2) [21].

NTDs are widespread in these regions. In 2014, Dr. Ricardo Fujiwara (a
professor at Brazil's Federal University of Minas Gerais) and I estimated
Brazil's contribution to the percentage of NTDs in the LAC region, with
most of that disease burden centered in Brazil's poorest northern states [21].
The numbers are impressive and demonstrate that Brazil is disproportionately plagued by NTDs. Despite the fact that Brazil accounts for approximately only one-third of the population in the LAC region, it accounts for
almost all of the region's schistosomiasis, kala-azar, leptospirosis, and leprosy, and more than one-third of the dengue fever, cutaneous leishmaniasis,
and malaria (table 8.2). By these estimates, Brazil is also responsible for approximately one-quarter of the region's people living with Chagas disease

Table 8.2. Brazil's burden of NTDs in the LAC region

Disease	% of LAC disease burden	Rank in the LAC region
Schistosomiasis	96	1
Kala-azar (visceral leishmaniasis)	93	1
Leptospirosis	92	1
Leprosy	86	1
Dengue	40	1
Cutaneous leishmaniasis	39	1
Malaria	36	1
Chagas disease	>25	2[a]
Intestinal helminth infections	24	1
Lymphatic filariasis	13	2
Onchocerciasis	2	5

Source: [21], doi:10.1016/J.micinf.2014.07.006.
[a] Our original estimate indicated that Brazil ranked ahead of Argentina in terms of the number of cases of Chagas disease in the LAC region.

and those who require treatment for intestinal helminth infections [21]. With the exception of onchocerciasis, Brazil ranks first or second in the Americas for each of the major NTDs. As explained earlier, these diseases trap people in poverty because of their chronic and debilitating effects and are therefore a key reason that Brazil's northeastern states cannot easily escape poverty. Just as Nigeria is ground zero for Africa's NTDs, the same could be said about Brazil in Latin America.

Brazil accounts for almost all of the schistosomiasis, kala-azar, leptospirosis, and leprosy in Latin America, and for more than one-third of the cases of dengue, cutaneous leishmaniasis, and malaria, ranking first among Latin American nations for these diseases.

The Brazilian Ministry of Health has not been oblivious to the problem of its NTDs and its links to poverty and in 2012 launched an Integrated Strategic Action Plan for eliminating several of these diseases through mass drug administration or, in the case of the intestinal helminth infections, reducing their overall "bioburden" [21]. Such activities are intimately tied to other poverty-reduction measures [22]. Prior to this period, Brazil's health activities were mostly decentralized and in the hands of state or municipal jurisdictions [21]. This decentralized feature made it difficult to eliminate NTDs that crossed state or municipal borders. A good example is LF in and around Recife in Pernambuco State, which should have been eliminated decades ago, but is only approaching elimination now. Of concern is whether the recent slowdown in Brazil's economy will derail or slow NTD control and elimination efforts.

Brazil is also in the grips of a severe dengue epidemic. All four dengue serotypes are now present in the country, and this creates a dangerous situation from a severe form of dengue, known as dengue hemorrhagic fever, that can result from an immune enhancement phenomena linked to past and current infection with different dengue strains. Since 2007, there has been an epidemic of severe pediatric dengue and dengue hemorrhagic fever in Brazil [23], and dengue is now hyperendemic in some large urban areas such as São Paulo, where all four dengue serotypes are present [24]. Prior to the 2014 FIFA World Cup, there were serious concerns that dengue epidemics could derail the games and local economies, especially in the tropical northeastern areas of the country [25]. Now a new arbovirus also threatens the nation. Zika virus emerged in Brazil in 2013 and expanded to create a massive epidemic post–FIFA World Cup; there are concerns that it is causing a significant level of congenital birth defects when it affects women during pregnancy [26].

Brazil is in the grips of a serious dengue epidemic, and Zika virus may be emerging simultaneously.

The nation is now facing serious threats from NTDs, some of which could contribute further to regional or economic slowdowns in the coming years. One of the bright spots for Brazil is its high level of innovation and ability to develop new drugs, diagnostics, and vaccines. A good example is CDTS, the Center for Technological Development in Health, based at the Oswaldo Cruz Foundation (FIOCRUZ), a new translational science and medicine institute headed by former FIOCRUZ president, Dr. Carlos Morel [27]. Brazil's two major vaccine manufacturers—FIOCRUZ Bio-Manguinhos and Instituto Butantan—now produce most of the vaccines needed for the country, and they are leading the development of new vaccines for dengue and other NTDs affecting the nation. Our Sabin Vaccine Institute PDP has been working with these organizations to develop NTD vaccines for the Americas—and eventually, worldwide, wherever NTDs are widespread. Thus, Brazil has the potential to provide part of the solution to a growing global innovation gap for new neglected disease technologies. I am particularly

On the bright side, Brazilian science is beginning to produce cutting-edge technologies for new drugs, diagnostics, and vaccines.

impressed with the quality of young Brazilian scientists. In our open access journal, *PLOS NTDs*, for example, Brazil ranks second behind only the United States in terms of the number of papers we receive from any single country.

Mexico

Mexico is the third G20 nation in Latin America, with a population of 124 million and an economy exceeding $1.2 trillion [1]. Economic growth since 2013 has been modest, as has been job growth and poverty reduction [28]. Almost 10% of the population, approximately 11 million people, are said to live in extreme poverty as defined by income levels adjusted for rural versus urban areas, in addition to not having access to one or more social rights [29]. Mexico also has a north-south poverty divide, with three contiguous states in southern Mexico—Chiapas, Guerrero, and Oaxaca—exhibiting some of the worst poverty and human development indices (fig. 8.3) [29]. But pov-

Figure 8.3.
Poverty in Mexico by state, 2010. Data from National Council for the Evaluation of Social Development Policy, *Report of Poverty in Mexico 2010: The Country, Its States and Its Municipalities* (Mexico City: CONEVAL, 2012).

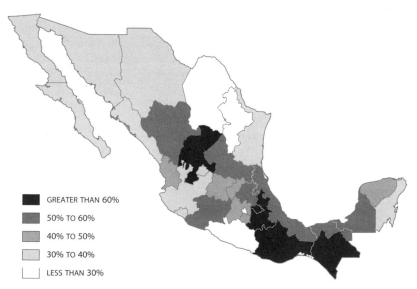

GREATER THAN 60%

50% TO 60%

40% TO 50%

30% TO 40%

LESS THAN 30%

erty is also common in some of the other southern provinces, including the Yucatán Peninsula in the Gulf of Mexico, where many Mayan villages are located [30].

NTDs are widespread amidst Mexico's extreme southern poverty. According to WHO, approximately 10 million Mexican children require regular deworming for their intestinal helminth infections [11], and neurocysticercosis, a parasitic worm infection of the brain and central nervous system, remains an important NTD [31, 32]. A study published in *PLOS NTDs* in 2012 reports that almost 150,000 people in Mexico suffer from epilepsy as a result of neurocysticercosis and approximately 100,000 have severe and chronic headaches [32]. However, Drs. Ana Flisser at Mexico's Universidad Nacional Autónoma de México (UNAM) and Dolores Correa at Mexico's Secretaria de Salud believe that the overall incidence of cysticercosis is now on the decline [33]. A form of cutaneous leishmaniasis similar to Aleppo evil, but caused by a different species, *Leishmania mexicana,* and transmitted by a different genus of *Lutzomyia* sandflies is also common. It is hyperendemic in Tabasco State, where it is linked to the region's cocoa industry [29].

Chagas disease is perhaps the worst NTD affecting Mexico. WHO has determined that almost one million people are infected with *T. cruzi* in Mexico [7], but alternative estimates indicate that this number may be several-fold higher [34]. For instance, UNAM's Drs. Alejandro Cruz-Reyes and José Miguel Pickering-López in their detailed analysis suggest that up to 5.9% of the Mexican population, around six million people, may actually be living with *T. cruzi* infection [35]. In some southern (and impoverished) Mexican states, the overall prevalence may be more than double the national average (fig. 8.4) [35]. The disease has also emerged as an important maternal and child health threat. WHO estimates that 185,000 women of reproductive age are infected with *T. cruzi*, while almost 2,000 cases of congenital Chagas disease occur annually as a result of pregnant women who pass their *T. cruzi* infection to their unborn fetus [7].

NTDs are widespread amidst Mexico's extreme southern poverty.

Still another major human tragedy is the barrier to treatment for the Mexican poor who suffer from Chagas disease and lack of access to either of the two essential medicines for the disease—benznidazole and nifurtimox. According to a study led by Harvard University's Dr. Michael Reich and published in *PLOS NTDs*, only 3,013 Chagas disease cases were registered nationally between the years 2007 and 2011,

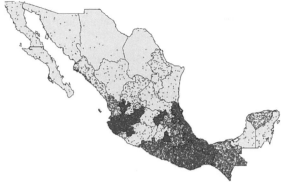

Figure 8.4.
Geographic distribution of Chagas disease in Mexico by
state. The points represent average density. From [35].

and in the year 2010–11 only 834 people were on antiparasitic treatment.
Overall, less than 0.5% of *T. cruzi* infected individuals receive treatment. The
Harvard group concluded that there needs to be "an increased commitment
to addressing this disease," in addition to adding antiparasitic medicines to
the national formulary, improving importation processes, educating health-
care providers, and providing improved and strengthened clinical guide-
lines [36]. An additional economic analysis of Chagas disease in Mexico
concluded that given the expense and long-term consequences of Chagasic
cardiomyopathy, it is ultimately less expensive to diagnose
and treat human *T. cruzi* infections than the current practice of "doing nothing" [37].

*Less than 1% of people
living with Chagas
disease in Mexico
have access to
diagnosis and
treatment.*

Such barriers to diagnosis and treatment and the lack
of available interventions for pregnant women to prevent
vertical transmission of Chagas disease reminded me very
much of the children living with HIV/AIDS, who faced a
similar situation in the early years of the AIDS epidemic
in the United States. I took care of many of these children as an attending
pediatrician in the pediatric HIV/AIDS clinic at Yale–New Haven Children's
Hospital during the 1990s. In 2012, I wrote an editorial asking whether Chagas disease might in some respects represent the "the new HIV/AIDS of
the Americas" [38]. The article generated a fair bit of controversy, and produced some pushback from the HIV/AIDS advocacy community, and even
some respected Chagas disease experts who objected to such comparisons.

However, I still think the comparisons have merit, particularly since most of the world's people living with Chagas disease remain undiagnosed, untreated, and unrecognized.

Finally, in Mexico dengue has emerged as an important public health problem, as it has in Brazil. A 2015 study led by Donald Shepard at Brandeis University found that 139,000 symptomatic episodes occurred in 2010–11, with costs averaging $170 million annually or about $1.56 per Mexican citizen [39].

Just as does Brazil, Mexico is also experiencing a serious dengue epidemic.

In response to a growing burden of disease and poverty from the NTDs and other conditions and the need for innovation to address these diseases, the family of Carlos Slim Helú, the Mexican telecommunications tycoon of Lebanese descent who ranks first or second as the world's wealthiest individual, has now established an important foundation (The Carlos Slim Foundation) in order to address the NTDs in Mexico and adjoining areas of Mesoamerica (Mexico and Central America). Led by Roberto Tapia Conyer, the Carlos Slim Foundation is supporting new and innovative approaches to NTD control in the region, especially dengue fever and Chagas disease. The Foundation is cosupporting the author's efforts to develop a therapeutic Chagas disease vaccine.

Mexico has a great potential to create innovative solutions for its NTDs. Among the major institutions are UNAM, as well as CINVESTAV, the nation's institute of advanced studies linked to its Instituto Politécnico Nacional. We are working closely with CINVESTAV scientists such as Dr. Jaime Ortega, who, together with Dr. Eric Dumonteil at the Universidad Autónoma de Yucatán, have important roles in developing our therapeutic Chagas disease vaccine.

Summary Points

1. Latin American countries exhibit some of the highest GINI indices or coefficients worldwide.
2. Approximately 130 million people living in the region are "chronically poor," including about 100 million who live on less than $2 per day.
3. Many of those poor live in Latin America's three wealthiest G20 countries—Argentina, Brazil, and Mexico, which account for 75% of

the region's economy, but also 95% of the cases of schistosomiasis, 61% of Chagas disease, 48% of intestinal helminth infections, and 42% of malaria cases.

4. In Argentina, most of the NTDs are found in the northern region, including the Argentine component of the Gran Chaco. The largest number of people living with Chagas disease can be found in Argentina. The nongovernmental organization Mundo Sano is working to reduce the NTD disease burden in these areas.

5. In Brazil, northeastern Brazil and the Amazon are the poorest regions and where most of the NTDs are found. Today, Brazil ranks first or second among Latin American countries in terms of the number of cases of at least 10 NTDs, including schistosomiasis, intestinal helminth infections, and dengue. Dengue fever and the Zika virus have emerged in many urban areas, where all four serotypes can be found, along with dengue hemorrhagic fever. Brazilian science functions at a high level, with a new translational science institute—CDTS FIOCRUZ—and the nation has great capacity to develop and test new vaccines through its FIOCRUZ Bio-Manguinhos and Instituto Butantan.

6. In Mexico, three contiguous states in the southern part of the country account for much of the nation's NTDs. Mexico has the world's largest number of congenital Chagas disease cases from mother-to-child transmission. Overall, less than 0.5% of people living with Chagas disease are diagnosed with the disease or have access to antiparasitic treatment. Dengue also has emerged as an important problem and is a serious drain on the Mexican economy, as is Chagas disease. The Carlos Slim Foundation is working to address some of these issues in the private nonprofit sector.

9 Australia, Canada, European Union, Russian Federation, and Turkey

Despite their modest populations, Australia (24 million people) and Canada (36 million people) represent two of the world's wealthiest economies, while the European Union has the single largest economy and a population exceeding 0.5 billion. The Russian Federation is geographically the biggest country, with a population approaching 150 million, and together with Turkey (75 million people) represents major emerging economies and important members of the G20.

Many people are surprised to learn that both extreme poverty and NTDs are also found in Australia and Canada, as well as the European countries and their immediate neighbors, Russia and Turkey. Each has pockets of impoverished people with important NTDs. However, for the most part, these diseases have not been systematically analyzed, and we have much more to learn.

Aboriginal Populations in Australia and Canada

Although both Australia and Canada are highly advanced and wealthy countries overall, each contains significant minorities living in poverty and affected by NTDs. Those populations are predominantly represented by aboriginal or indigenous populations. Globally, aboriginal groups constitute approximately 5% of the population—almost 400 million people. These groups are especially prone to NTDs and poverty, especially rural poverty, and together account for about 15% of the world's impoverished population. Extreme poverty and the associated factors of inadequate housing and access to health care, living in degraded environments with low levels of sanitation and nutrition, and forced migrations, are among the factors that contribute to the high prevalence of NTDs among aboriginal groups [1]. Such conditions bear some similarities to populations fleeing conflict areas and living in postconflict settings. In addition, aboriginal populations have been shown to often suffer from high rates of NCDs owing to excessive tobacco use and consumption of alcohol or other substances [1].

Australia. The estimated 500,000 Aboriginal Australians are highly vulnerable to some important NTDs [1, 2]. Their diseases include intestinal helminth infections such as hookworm infection and strongyloidiasis, not unlike the occurrence of those same diseases among populations living in northern Argentina. In the case of human *Strongyloides* infections, there is also a link in Australia to coinfections with a retrovirus known as human T-lymphotropic virus 1 (HTLV-1) [1, 2].

Ectoparasitic infestation with the mite *Sarcoptes scabei* is also an important yet neglected health issue among Aboriginal Australians, with the prevalence exceeding 10% in northern Australia [3, 4]. Scabies is associated with a characteristic rash that can be intensely itchy as a result of mites burrowing into the skin (fig. 9.1). Hyperinfestation with the scabies mite, a condition known as crusted or Norwegian scabies, can occur and result in severe disfigurement and fissuring of the skin [3]. The condition is highly debilitating and, like many NTDs, can also result in social stigma or exclusion. Both scabies and crusted scabies can also lead to secondary *Streptococcus* and *Staphylococcus* bacterial infections, with the former causing either rheumatic heart disease or glomerulonephritis, a kidney disease that can lead to renal failure.

Figure 9.1.
Hand of an adolescent girl exhibiting scabies infestation with typical secondary bacterial infection. From [4].

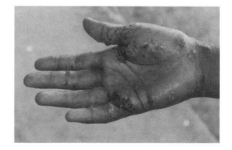

Finally, blinding trachoma is another important bacterial NTD, as is melioidosis [4, 5]. As regards the former, Australia is currently the world's only high-income country with endemic trachoma [6]. It is also the only high-income country with endemic Buruli ulcer [7].

NTDs are widespread among Australia's Aboriginal populations. Australia is currently the only high-income country with endemic trachoma, Buruli ulcer, scabies, and other NTDs.

In Australia, mass drug administration could have an important role in reducing the burden of NTDs among Aboriginal populations. Three drugs in particular show promise: ivermectin, albendazole, and azithromycin. Potentially, MDA with ivermectin in combination with albendazole could be used for controlling strongyloidiasis and hookworm coinfections. Moreover, ivermectin MDA may have collateral benefits for the control of scabies in Australia [8], and an International Alliance for the Control of Scabies (IACS) has been established for assessing the global impact of both the disease and opportunities for MDA approaches [4]. Similarly, MDA with azithromycin could help to eliminate blinding trachoma from Australia [1, 6].

Canada. It comes as a surprise to many that the frozen regions of Arctic could host NTDs, but indigenous people (such as the estimated 150,000 Inuit) living in this region, including the Canadian Arctic, frequently suffer from these infections [1, 9]. Many of the Arctic NTDs are parasitic zoonoses acquired from inadequately cooked meat [1, 9–11]. Walruses and seals, for example are major sources of a unique type of trichinellosis, a serious parasitic helminth infection of the muscles caused by *Trichinella spiralis nativa*. Two forms of human echinococcosis are also present, both acquired from dogs, and although still a rare disease, they can result in significant health-care expenditures [10]. Toxoplasmosis is another parasitic zoonosis from wild game and hunting [11]. A recent surveillance study conducted among more than 200 volunteers in northern Saskatchewan found that 65% were seropositive for at least one parasite, mostly those highlighted above [12].

Zoonotic NTDs are highly endemic in the Canadian Arctic, especially among the Inuit and other indigenous groups. Climate change may promote the further emergence of additional NTDs.

There is a need to expand surveillance activities on the zoonotic NTDs of the Canadian Arctic and to conduct studies to improve our understanding of the ecology and transmission dynamics of these diseases. Community health education campaigns on the infection risks from hunting and food consumption would also be helpful [13], along with improved communications between the human and veterinary public health communities to combat the zoonotic NTDs of the region.

Possibly more than any other geographic area, the Arctic and Canadian Arctic are disproportionately affected by the forces linked to climate change [13, 14]. A circumpolar working group has convened and identified a group of parasitic and zoonotic infections as likely candidates to increase in prevalence as a consequence of climate change, including those highlighted above, in addition to some bacterial NTDs such as anthrax, leptospirosis, and tularemia and viral NTDs including West Nile virus infection, tick-borne encephalitis, and hantavirus infection [14]. Outside of the circumpolar region, *Leptospira* have been identified among inner-city rats in Vancouver [15], such that leptospirosis and other NTDs may also be found among poorer populations in Canada.

European Union

The EU comprises 28 countries and has a combined population of just more than 500 million people. At approximately $18.5 trillion, the EU also represents almost one-quarter of the global economy [16]. Since the end of 2009, a debt crisis, mostly affecting five EU member states (all but four in southern Europe)—Cyprus, Greece, Ireland, Portugal, and Spain—has threatened the economic stability of the EU. As of this writing, the potential default of Greece's debt has reached crisis proportions.

In western Europe, based on paleoparasitology evidence from World War I and other human remains, NTDs, including intestinal helminth infections, were once widespread [17]. Even today, certain NTDs are still present, such as enterobiasis among Norwegian children [18], and there is evidence for the emergence of two major zoonotic helminthiases: neurocysticercosis and echinococcosis [19–21]. However, most of Europe's NTDs are concentrated in its underbelly of poverty in eastern Europe, and especially its southeastern region (fig. 9.2) [22]. The Balkan nations (Albania, Bosnia and Herzegovina, Bulgaria, Croatia, Kosovo, Macedonia, Montenegro, Romania, and Serbia) are still emerging from devastating wars and forced human migrations during the 1990s, which damaged both health systems and educational infrastructure. Intestinal parasites, including helminth infections (e.g., as-

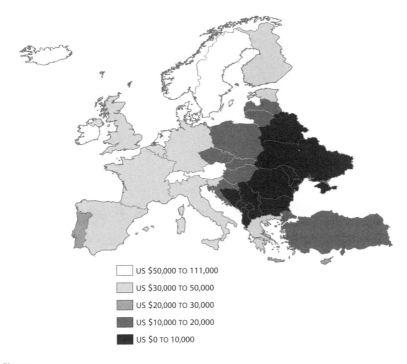

Figure 9.2.
West-to-east poverty gradient map of Europe, showing 2014 GDP per capita.
Derived from data at http://data.worldbank.org/indicator/NY.GDP.PCAP.CD.

cariasis, trichuriasis, and enterobiasis) and protozoan infections, are still prevalent in rural areas of these countries [22–24], as are the major zoonotic helminth infections—cysticercosis, echinococcosis, tae-niasis [25–30] and zoonotic bacterial infections—brucel-losis and leptospirosis.

Zoonotic NTDs are commonly found among the poor living in the Balkans and elsewhere in southeastern Europe.

In both southeastern and southern Europe, there are serious concerns about the reemergence of dengue after a more than 50-year absence, with a 2012 dengue outbreak occurring on the Portuguese archipelago of Madeira [31], in addition to new cases or outbreaks of West Nile virus infection [32, 33], chikungunya [34], and Crimean-Congo hemorrhagic fever [35], among others. Strongyloidiasis is still present in rural areas of Spain and France [36, 37], and recently opisthorchiasis (liver fluke) has emerged in Italy [38], while schistosomiasis has appeared in Corsica [39].

*Arboviral infections
and other NTDs,
including fluke
infections, are
emerging in southern
Europe. There is a
risk that vivax
malaria might also
reemerge. Poverty is
a key factor, but
climate change may
also play a role.*

Chagas disease imported from Latin America is common in Spain [40], and visceral leishmaniasis is endemic there, where it is also an important opportunistic infection of people living with HIV/AIDS [41]. Additional vulnerable populations in the EU include the Roma, a group of 7–9 million people based mostly in central and eastern Europe who face high levels of poverty and unemployment, and the many immigrants from Africa fleeing extreme poverty and conflict [22].

Overall, there is a need to better collect and disseminate data on Europe's NTDs, as well as to initiate efforts to conduct active surveillance. With regard to the arboviral infections, it has been proposed that the NTDs now emerging in southern Europe could spread into northwestern Europe or elsewhere across the continent [42]. In 2013, we proposed the establishment of an institute or center devoted to such activities and recommended Greece as a potential home [43]. The rationale for situating such activities in Greece is that the country is now a highly vulnerable region for NTDs, owing to its poverty linked to national debt, and also that it is located near the confluence of southeastern Europe's NTDs and those emerging from Africa and the Middle East (table 9.1) [43]. At the same time, it has a historically strong track record in biotechnology and scientific investigation.

In the meantime, a European Centre for Disease Prevention and Control (ECDC) established in 2004 and based in Sweden has recently created a European Environment and Epidemiology (E3) Network to monitor the emergence of some key NTDs affecting the region. The E3 Network has identified areas of potential vivax malaria transmission and malaria reemergence in Greece [44]. Prior to World War II, malaria was widespread in Greece and was a driving force that thwarted economic development [45].

Overall, there appears to be a troublesome and recent rise in NTDs in southern Europe. Within the past few years, we have seen the emergence or reemergence of several arboviral infections, vivax malaria, and schistosomiasis, as well as others. Is there a common theme that might explain these findings? In a 2015 article in the *Washington Post*, I wrote that there are several possibilities, including the recent economic downturns in Greece, Spain, Italy, and elsewhere, and evidence that climate change is now affecting this region [46]. Still another factor might be linked to human migra-

Table 9.1. Major NTDs of Europe and the MENA region

NTDs	Europe	MENA region
Parasitic infections		
Ascariasis/trichuriasis	+	+
Toxocariasis	+	+
Fascioliasis	+	+
Schistosomiasis	+	+
Taeniasis	+	+
Trichinellosis	+	−
Echinococcosis	−	+
Leishmaniasis	+	+
Toxoplasmosis	+	+
Vivax malaria	+	+
Bacterial/viral infections		
Brupcellosis	+	+
Leptospirosis	+	+
Chikungunya virus	+	+
Crimean-Congo hemorrhagic fever	+	+
Dengue	+	+
Rift Valley fever	−	+

Source: [43], modified to include new evidence of schistosomiasis in Corsica, doi:10.1371/journal.pntd.0001757.t001.

tions of people fleeing ISIS-occupied areas in Libya, Iraq, and Syria [46]. Each of these factors needs to be investigated in more detail.

Russian Federation and Turkey

The World Bank projects a mostly negative forecast for the Russian economy in the coming years as a result of deep-rooted structural problems, sanctions, falling oil prices (Russia's major export), and diminished investments [47]. Poverty reductions that occurred over the past decade in the Putin era are expected to reverse in Russia's new contracting economy, with some projections indicating that 20 million Russians (out of a total population of 142 million) will live below the poverty line [48]. The NTDs possibly arising from this situation, together with climate change, remains unclear, although it might include the reemergence of malaria [49] or West Nile virus infection [50]. Currently, three parasitic zoonoses are still important NTDs in the Russian Federation. They include several forms of hydatid disease (both cystic and alveolar echinococcosis) [51], diphyllobothriasis [52], and liver fluke infection caused by *Opisthorchis felineus* [53, 54]. Russian opisthorchiasis is centered in its western Siberian region, where it is highly endemic and causes bile duct carcinoma [53, 54]. A related infection caused by *Metorchis bilis* is also a significant liver fluke infection.

Turkey's economy now exceeds $750 billion, and according to the World Bank, in less than a decade its per capita income has tripled, exceeding that of many of its MENA neighbors [55]. The EU remains Turkey's largest economic partner and is responsible for almost one-half of its trade [55]. As of 2011, only 2.6% of its population of 75 million lived on less than $2 per day [56]. Vivax malaria is the only autochthonous form of the disease, but the number of cases has been declining [57], whereas cutaneous leishmaniasis, known locally as Urfa boil, Antep boil, Halep boil, or oriental sore, and caused by both *Leishmania tropica* and *L. infantum*, is still widespread, especially among the poor [58]. Intestinal parasitic infections are also on the decline, especially in urban areas, where the economy is more robust [59], while echinococcosis remains an important NTD in rural areas [60]. Brucellosis is believed to be an important zoonotic bacterial NTD that remains underdiagnosed [61]. Arboviruses, including West Nile virus and Crimean-Congo hemorrhagic fever, are emerging here, as they are in southern Europe [62, 63]. The epidemiology of each of these NTDs is changing rapidly because of the widespread refugee influx from ISIS-occupied Syria and Iraq. According to the United Nations High Commission on Refugees, the largest contingent of emigrants from Syria—1.8 million people—has entered Turkey [64]. It can therefore be expected that the number of total NTDs affecting Turkey may rise in the coming years.

Concluding Remarks

NTDs remain important diseases among aboriginal groups in Australia and Canada. In Europe, the Russian Federation, and Turkey, parasitic and zoonotic NTDs are still commonly found among the poor, but there is also a new reality. Arboviral infections and other vector-borne infections are emerging in these areas as a consequence of new poverty, especially in southern Europe and Russia, together with climate change, and possibly the arrival of some displaced populations from the Middle East and North Africa.

Summary Points

1. The NTDs in Australia and Canada are important among aboriginal populations.
   a. Aboriginal Australians are affected by hookworm infection and strongyloidiasis, as well as scabies and its bacterial complications leading to rheumatic heart disease and chronic renal disease. Trachoma is also endemic.
   b. Zoonotic and foodborne parasitic infections such as trichinellosis, echinococcosis, and toxoplasmosis are major NTDs among aboriginal populations living in the Arctic region, including the Canadian Arctic. Climate change and global warming are expected to exacerbate the incidence of these diseases in the coming years.
2. The European Union is the largest economy, but NTDs remain widespread in areas of poverty in eastern and southern Europe.
   a. In eastern Europe, intestinal parasites, including ascariasis, enterobiasis, and giardiasis, are still common, as are zoonotic infections—brucellosis, cysticercosis, and echinococcosis.
   b. In southern Europe, key arboviral infections are emerging or reemerging, including dengue fever and West Nile virus infection, in addition to a number of parasitic infections such as strongyloidiasis, opisthorchiasis, schistosomiasis, and leishmaniasis. Vivax malaria also has the potential to emerge in Greece and elsewhere.
3. The Russian Federation economy is contracting, and NTDs can be expected to reappear in this setting. Opisthorchiasis is a serious foodborne trematodiasis linked to cholangiocarcinoma.
4. Turkey is at risk for reemerging NTDs coming across the border from ISIS-occupied areas in Syria and Iraq.
5. Overall, there is an extreme dearth of surveillance, prevalence, and incidence data on NTDs in Europe and adjoining areas in Russia and Turkey.

United States of America

The finding of widespread NTDs among the poor in the United States was driven home almost literally as I took time to drive around some of the most impoverished areas of Texas, including Houston's Fifth Ward. But even prior to my relocating to the Texas Medical Center in 2011, it was clear that NTDs have an intimate connection to poverty, including a significant but largely hidden level of poverty in the United States.

In a 2006 paper published in the journal, *Vaccine* [1], and a subsequent article in the *Lancet* [2], we began to identify how NTDs not only occurred in the setting of poverty, but also were a major cause of poverty among the bottom billion. Notable among those effects were how NTDs reinforced poverty because of their long-term and deleterious effects on child development, intelligence, and cognition; the worker productivity of adults; and the health of girls and women, especially in pregnancy [1, 2]. NTDs and poverty were linked at the hip. It became increasingly clear that if you wanted to find NTDs, all you needed to do was to look for extreme poverty—and there they were.

NTDs can be found wherever you encounter extreme poverty.

The Other America

It was then I remembered a book I had read decades ago either in junior high school or high school titled *The Other America: Poverty in the United States* written by the social activist Michael Harrington, who in 1962 highlighted the hidden burden of poverty in an otherwise prosperous post–World War II America [3]. He ventured into America's inner cities, the Mississippi Delta, Appalachia, and rural California, where migrant farmworkers toiled, to eloquently describe millions of lives seldom viewed from our major highways and roads. His book was instrumental in convincing President Lyndon B. Johnson and his administration to launch the war on poverty, inaugurated with the president's landmark State of the Union address in 1964.

Years later, when I was a full professor, I found a torn and yellowed paperback copy of Harrington's book. His opening paragraphs in the introductory chapter, titled "The Invisible America," had a powerful effect:

There is a familiar America. It is celebrated in speeches and advertised on television and in the magazines. It has the highest mass standard of living the world has ever known. . . . While this discussion was carried on, there existed another America. In it dwelt somewhere between 40,000,000 and 50,000,000 citizens of the land. They were poor. They still are. To be sure, the other America is not impoverished in the same sense as those poor nations where millions cling to hunger as a defense against starvation. This country has escaped such extremes. That does not change the fact that tens of millions of Americans are, at this very moment, maimed in body and spirit, existing at levels beneath those necessary for human decency. If these people are not starving, they are hungry, and sometimes fat with hunger, for that is what cheap foods do. They are without adequate housing and education and medical care [3].

Harrington's words and message inspired me to begin a profound examination of poverty in the United States. According to the US Census Bureau, as of 2013, approximately 45.3 million people lived at or below the poverty line [4], roughly the same number as in Harrington's *Other America*. However, back in 1962 that number was equivalent to almost one-quarter of the US population, whereas today it represents 14.5%. The poverty threshold set by the US government is a dollar amount for total yearly income for a family of four—currently between

The new face of poverty in America: Today, 20 million Americans live in extreme poverty, and 1.65 million families in the United States live on less than $2 per day.

$20,000 and $30,000, which is based on a complicated array of parameters adjusted for inflation and other factors.

I concede that most of the 45.3 million Americans living below the poverty line do not face the same desperate circumstances as the poorest people living in, say, China or Indonesia who live on less than $2 per day. Instead, with respect to America's NTDs, I am concerned about the following two statistics:

- The first is from the National Center for Poverty at the University of Michigan, where H. L. Shaefer and K. Edin report that 1.65 million American households, with 3.55 million children, live in extreme poverty in a given month, meaning on less than $2 per day, per person [5]. In other words, there are at least 4–5 million people living at the level of extreme poverty—indeed similar to what we might find in China or Indonesia, or anywhere else globally.
- An almost equally compelling statistic is the finding in 2011 that 20.5 million Americans live at or below one-half of the US poverty level, another metric of extreme poverty [6]. I sometimes refer to this group as America's "bottom 20 million." Such recalcitrant poverty was an inspiration for the journalist and author Sasha Abramsky to write a follow-up book, *The American Way of Poverty: How the Other Half Still Lives* [7].

In this setting of extreme poverty, NTDs flourish in the United States, just as they do across the blue marble. Furthermore, just as poverty among the G20 countries is concentrated in selected areas of each of the constituent nations, American poverty is also focused in specific regions. American poverty also disproportionately affects specific ethnic groups.

NTDs flourish in this new American poverty.

The Ethnogeography of America's "Bottom 20 Million"

According to the US Census Bureau, both non-Hispanic blacks and those of Hispanic origin suffer from as much as three times higher rates of poverty than non-Hispanic whites. Native American groups in the United States also experience crushing poverty. These rates are even higher among subsets of those racial/ethnic groups; for example, almost one-half of black or

Table 10.1. Rank of US states by poverty rates

	Poverty rate	Rank among US states
Mississippi	21.0	1
New Mexico	19.9	2
Arizona	19.1	3
District of Columbia	19.1	3
Louisiana	18.9	5
Georgia	18.5	6
Texas	17.7	7

Source: [9], doi:10.1371/journal.pntd.0003012.t001.
Note: Percentage of people in poverty by state using three-year averages, 2009–11 (http://www.census
.gov/hhes/www/poverty/data/incpovhlth/2011/tables.html).

Hispanic single female householders with children under the age of 18 live
in poverty [8]. Indeed, as shown in table 10.1, the southern states with high
levels of black or Hispanic poverty constitute those with the highest poverty
rates in America, led by (in order) Mississippi, New Mexico, Arizona, District of Columbia, Louisiana, Georgia, and Texas [9]. Texas is the largest of
those states in terms of numbers of impoverished people—out of a total
population now exceeding 27 million, almost 5 million
Texans live in poverty. This finding provided a rationale
for my locating the National School of Tropical Medicine
in Texas.

> *We established the
> National School of
> Tropical Medicine in
> Texas because it is
> the state with some
> of the largest
> numbers of people
> who live in poverty.*

The identification of Texas and adjoining southern
states as the home of American poverty, and ultimately
NTDs, does not tell the full story. For instance, two social
scientists, A. K. Glasmeier and J. B. Holt, independently
identified distressed regions of extreme poverty in America [10, 11]. As shown in figure 10.1 in maps produced by
Holt, the following six major regions were identified: the Mississippi Delta
and adjoining border regions of the American South ("Cotton Belt"), Appalachia, the border region with Mexico, Native American tribal lands of the
American Southwest and northern Great Plains, disadvantaged (and highly
segregated) urban areas of the northeast, and the "Rust Belt" [10, 11].

Yet another approach to looking at the ethnogeography of poverty in
America was developed by Dr. Christopher Murray and his colleagues in

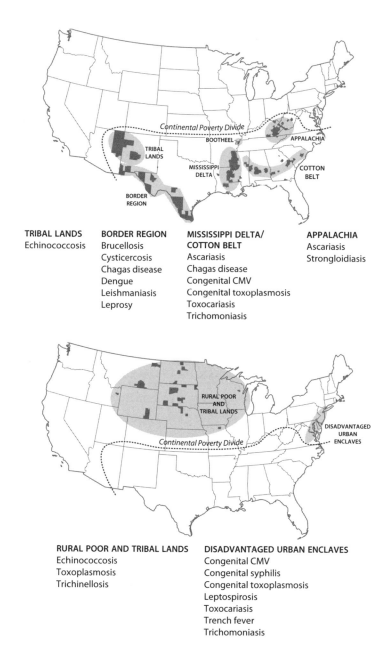

Figure 10.1.

Location of US counties that represent spatial clusters in which poverty rates are at least two standard deviations higher than the national mean. *Top:* Counties south of the Continental Divide. *Bottom:* Counties north of the Continental Divide. From [11].

2005, who identified "eight Americas" based on distinct epidemiologic patterns, including four associated with both higher mortality and poverty: poor whites living in Appalachia, Native Americans living on reservations in the West, poor blacks living in the rural South, and blacks living in high-risk urban environments [12]. The paradigm of NTDs linked to extreme poverty in these four to six regions helped me to create a framework to search for American NTDs.

NTDs are diseases of extreme poverty: America's NTDs can be found predominantly in specific geographic regions where poverty is rampant and among specific ethnic/racial groups who disproportionately suffer from extreme poverty.

America's Leading NTDs

In 2008, I published my first analysis of NTDs in the areas where America's "bottom 20 million" who live in extreme poverty are found [8]. The search relied on the US National Center for Biotechnology Information's PubMed biomedical literature database, which in a few cases reported previously published estimates of the number of cases of each NTD. However, for most of the NTDs there were no published national estimates. In such cases, I provided a range of estimates based on reported prevalence rates of a given NTD among a selected community and then extrapolated an overall prevalence number based on a population's likelihood of having similar socioeconomic, racial, or ethnic demographics. In some cases, Chris Murray's population estimates for the four impoverished Americas provided the population at risk number.

My initial estimates are shown in table 10.2. Among African Americans living in poverty in the American South or inner-city areas were figured to be hundreds of thousands or even millions of cases of selected NTDs, such as toxocariasis, and trichomoniasis, as well as congenital syphilis and cytomegalovirus infection [8]. Among Hispanics living in poverty in Texas and elsewhere were up to one million cases of Chagas disease and tens of thousands of cases of cysticercosis and dengue fever [8]. Strongyloidiasis is prevalent among poor whites living Appalachia [8].

The finding of high prevalence rates of NTDs among non-Hispanic populations was especially important. As I began to write and speak more about widespread NTDs

America's NTDs go way beyond importation through immigration. Instead, we have widespread transmission of NTDs among the poor.

Table 10.2. Initial estimate of NTD prevalence in the United States

Neglected disease category	Disease	Estimated number of cases	Major regions or populations at risk
Soil-transmitted helminth infections	Ascariasis	<4 million	Appalachia, American South
	Toxocariasis	1.3–2.8 million	Inner cities, American South, Appalachia
	Strongyloidiasis	68,000–100,000	Appalachia, African refugees
	Trichinellosis	16 (insufficient data)	Arctic Alaska
Platyhelminth infections	Cysticercosis	41,400–169,000	US-Mexico borderlands
	Schistosomiasis	8,000	African refugees
	Echinococcosis	Insufficient data	Tribal lands and Arctic Alaska
Protozoan infections	Giardiasis	2.0–2.5 million	All regions
	Trichomoniasis	880,000 (black women)	American South, inner cities
	Cryptosporidiosis	300,000	All regions
	Chagas disease	3,000 to >1 million	US-Mexico borderlands, American South
	Cyclosporiasis	16,624	All regions
	Congenital toxoplasmosis	≤4,000 annually	American South, inner cities, US-Mexico borderlands, Arctic Alaska
	Leishmaniasis	Insufficient data	US-Mexico borderlands
	Amebiasis	Insufficient data	US-Mexico borderlands
Bacterial infections	Congenital syphilis	1,528 between 2000 and 2002	American South, inner cities
	Brucellosis	1,554	US-Mexico borderlands
	Bovine tuberculosis	129 cases between 1994 and 2000	US-Mexico borderlands
	Leprosy	166	US-Mexico borderlands
	Trench fever	Insufficient data	Inner cities
	Leptospirosis	Insufficient data	Inner cities
Viral infections	Dengue fever	110,000–200,000 new infections annually	US-Mexico borderlands, American South
	Congenital cytomegalovirus	27,002 annually; 6,652 in blacks; 4,196 in Hispanics	American South, inner cities
	Human rabies	2	All regions

Source: [8], doi:10.1371/journal.pntd.0000256.t002.

among the poor in America, many—especially those from the conservative right—were quick to blame immigration from Mexico and El Salvador. Instead, as I pointed out in a 2012 op-ed piece published in the *New York Times*, while immigration could explain some of America's NTDs, most in fact were acquired within US borders, and transmission was linked to extreme poverty [13].

The NTDs are not rare diseases in the United States. In fact, they are widespread but hidden among the unseen poor and commonly mistaken for other conditions.

My first attempt to best determine the true prevalence of the major NTDs in the United States was hampered by a general absence of detailed knowledge about the incidence for these diseases. I was especially struck by the dearth of active surveillance studies. When I began, almost no one was looking for the NTDs in America. Actively looking for NTDs is critical because, just like NTDs abroad, most of them are chronic and debilitating conditions that can mimic NCDs. For example, unless you actively pursue a diagnosis of Chagas disease by using a specific test, a patient's heart disease could be ascribed to some other cause. The same is true for an individual's epilepsy or neurocognitive delays from cysticercosis or toxocariasis that might be mistaken for some other neurologic illness. The initial evidence, however, I felt made a compelling case that while the NTDs are mostly hidden, they are actually widespread in the United States. Based on such observations in 2008, my initial policy recommendation was to call on federal, state, and local public health officials to pursue programs of active surveillance for these diseases.

My initial estimates led to two key policy recommendations: (1) pursue programs of active surveillance for NTDs, and (2) conduct studies to understand how NTDs are transmitted within US borders.

Another important need was to better understand how these diseases are transmitted. While some assumed that these NTDs were imported through immigration from our southern border with Mexico, in many cases there was preliminary evidence for transmission within US borders. A good example was Chagas disease, which subsequently was shown to be widespread among dogs in the state of Texas. Clearly, the dogs were not slipping in from Mexico and Central America.

Subsequently, we began working with the US Centers for Disease Control and Prevention (CDC) to obtain a more accurate accounting of NTDs in the nation [14]. Captain Monica Parise, MD, of the US Public Health Service heads the Parasitic Disease Branch at CDC; her boss, Dr. Larry Slutsker, oversaw both NTDs and a large malaria portfolio prior to retirement. Shown in table 10.3 is a refined estimate of the neglected parasitic infections in the United States, which accounts for most of the American NTDs. In all, I estimate that 12 million Americans live with a neglected parasitic infection.

It is likely that 12 million Americans live with an NTD in the United States.

The bottom line is that NTDs are not rare diseases in the United States. A specific description of each of the major NTDs follows:

Toxocariasis is a parasitic worm infection acquired from dogs and cats. Many stray dogs and cats are infected with their own version of *Ascaris* roundworms known as *Toxocara canis* and *T. cati*, respectively. Infected dogs and cats harbor millions of parasite eggs in their feces. Dog and cat feces released into the environment subsequently contaminate sandboxes, playgrounds, and other environmental surfaces. Driving through poor areas of Houston and elsewhere in Texas and the American South, I am struck by the frequent sight of stray dogs, often traveling in packs. There are so many eggs that they are practically ubiquitous in areas of environmental degradation, including play areas across poor urban and rural landscapes. Children playing outdoors come into contact with microscopic *Toxocara* eggs. The eggs are ingested, and they hatch in their intestinal tract. The released larvae migrate to the children's lungs, where they can cause wheezing and pulmonary damage, or to their brains, where the larvae can cause seizures, but also cognitive and developmental delays. I believe that toxocariasis is the most common helminth infection in the United States [15]. Based on CDC studies showing a high prevalence of toxocariasis among African Americans living in poverty [16], I estimate that up to 2.8 million of this population may be infected with either *T. canis* or *T. cati* [8, 9]. Additional studies from Drs. M. G. Walsh and M. A. Haseeb at SUNY Downstate Medical Center in Brooklyn have linked human toxocariasis to lung and neurologic dysfunction [17, 18]. Their work led me to ask whether this NTD could partly be responsible for the achievement gap noted among socioeconomically disadvantaged children in inner-city or poor rural schools [19]. Unfortunately, toxocariasis remains terribly understudied, and largely unrecognized by the major US government agencies. In a recent systematic review, we found only 18 studies from North America with original prevalence, incidence, or case data for toxocariasis [20].

Table 10.3. Neglected parasitic infections in the United States

Neglected parasitic infection	Selected prevalence data	Major risk factors	Clinical sequelae in adults and children[a]	Clinical sequelae in adults and children[a]	Congenital clinical sequelae
Toxocariasis	>21% seroprevalence among African-Americans (up to 2.8 million African-Americans); >17% seroprevalence in the American South	African-American race, male sex, poverty, low education level, lead ingestion, contact with dogs, coinfection with *Toxoplasma*	Neurologic and psychiatric: cognitive delays, epilepsy, ocular manifestations	Pulmonary: diminished lung function asthma	Not well established
Cysticercosis	Up to 41,000–169,000 infected persons; likely widely underrecognized, with only an estimated 1,000 hospitalized cases diagnosed	Hispanic immigrants	Neurologic: epilepsy, chronic headaches	None	Not well established
Chagas disease	300,167 cases	Hispanic-Americans	Cardiovascular: cardiomyopathy neurysms; conduction disturbances; sudden death	Gastrointestinal: megaviscera	Congenital Chagas disease syndrome
Toxoplasmosis	1.1 million new cases annually, including 21,505 cases of ocular toxoplasmosis and up to 4,000 cases of congenital toxoplasmosis	African-American ethnicity and poverty	Neurologic and psychiatric: cerebritis, schizophrenia, bipolar and other mood disorders	Ocular: retinitis and retinal scars, other ocular findings	Congenital toxoplasmosis syndrome: hydrocephalus, chorioretinitis, intracranial calcifications, cognitive deficits, hearing loss
Trichomoniasis	7.4 million new cases annually	African-American ethnicity (10 times more common)	Genitourinary: vaginitis, pelvic inflammatory disease, pregnancy complications	HIV coinfections	Neonatal infections
Total	Approximately 12 million incident or prevalent infections, including some people living with chronic sequelae				

Source: [9], doi:10.1371/journal.pntd.0003012.t002.

[a] Features that produce clinical manifestations and sequelae similar to selected noncommunicable diseases.

Other soil-transmitted helminth infections, ascariasis and hookworm infection, were once widespread but were almost eliminated following economic reforms and New Deal legislation in the 1930s that helped to urbanize and transform the workforce as factory and other industrial jobs came to replace agrarian activities. However, Dr. Rojelio Mejia from the National School of Tropical Medicine, working with social activist Catherine Flowers, has found soon to be published evidence that these infections may still remain in rural Alabama and elsewhere in the American South.

Cysticercosis is another parasitic helminth infection affecting the human brain and an important cause of seizures and epilepsy, especially among Hispanic populations in Texas and elsewhere in the United States. The disease results from ingesting the eggs found in the feces of humans infected with the pork tapeworm *Taenia solium*. Adult tapeworm *T. solium* infections occur commonly in many parts of Latin America, Africa, and Asia where pigs have access to infected human feces. Individuals who harbor these tapeworms shed eggs, which can be transmitted to household contacts. Egg ingestion results in larval tapeworms appearing in the brain and muscles, which can trigger seizures and epilepsy [21]. I estimate that between 41,000 and 169,000 individuals in the United States have cysticercosis [8, 9], but these numbers need refinement based on urgently needed surveillance studies.

Chagas disease is caused by microscopic, single-celled protozoan parasites known as trypanosomes. *Trypanosoma cruzi* can invade the heart tissue to produce a serious and debilitating heart infection known as Chagasic cardiomyopathy. The disease is transmitted by kissing bugs, also known as triatomines. The CDC in studies currently led by Drs. Susan Montgomery and Caryn Bern (now at the University of California, San Francisco) estimates that approximately 300,000 people in the United States live with Chagas disease, most of whom are immigrants from poor regions of Latin America, including Argentina, Brazil, Mexico, and adjoining regions of Central America, where the disease is highly endemic [22]. However, Drs. Kristy O. Murray and Melissa Nolan Garcia from our National School of Tropical Medicine at Baylor College of Medicine have been conducting extensive studies in Texas to demonstrate a significant level of autochthonous infection, meaning infection acquired in Texas, especially southeastern Texas [23–26]. Of note, almost one half of *T. cruzi*-infected individuals who were identified by blood screening were found to have evidence of Chagasic cardiomyopathy [24]. They also identified some Chagas disease patients who might have acquired their infections through outdoor activities such as hunting and camping [26]. Another important factor for Chagas disease in Texas is the finding that many dogs are also infected with *T. cruzi*. Dr. Sarah Hamer and her colleagues at the Texas A&M University School of Veterinary Medicine found that the overall seroprevalence of Chagas disease among shelter dogs across different regions of Texas was almost 9%, but in some shelters, such as in the San Antonio area, the seroprevalence was as high as 14% [27]. I believe that, in terms of understanding the full extent of the Chagas disease problem in Texas, we are seeing merely the tip of the iceberg—or, as we once indicated at a Houston conference on NTDs, "the ears of the armadillo" [28].

Toxoplasmosis is another serious protozoan and zoonotic infection acquired either from ingesting the infective stages found in cat feces or in undercooked meats. The CDC's finding that many individuals are simultaneously infected with *Toxocara* and *Toxoplasma* suggests that the cat may be an important source for both infections [29]. In addition, the CDC, in studies led by Dr. J. L. Jones, has determined that more than one million new cases of toxoplasmosis occur annually, with those living in poverty at greatest risk [30, 31]. Toxoplasmosis is a leading cause of eye disease in the United States, resulting in a condition known as chorioretinitis, as well as congenital disease transmitted from mother to child [31]. Drs. Robert Yolken and E. F. Torrey and their colleagues at Johns Hopkins University School of Medicine have argued that toxoplasmosis is a serious condition that can lead to schizophrenia and other psychiatric illnesses [19, 32], although this hypothesis requires more extensive and confirmatory studies.

Trichomoniasis is a sexually transmitted protozoan infection caused by *Trichomonas vaginalis* that affects more than seven million Americans [33], although other estimates indicate about one-half as many infections occur annually [34]. African American women are disproportionately affected by as much as 10-fold [35]. The *T. vaginalis* parasite is an important cofactor in the American HIV/AIDS epidemic, as it is linked to increased viral shedding and transmission [36, 37].

Arboviral infections. In addition to the 12 million Americans affected by neglected parasitic infections are many more who suffer from the arboviral infections transmitted mostly by mosquitoes. Texas and the Gulf Coast host two species of *Aedes* mosquitoes—*Aedes aegypti* and *Ae. albopictus*—that are capable of transmitting dengue fever as well as chikungunya and Zika virus infections. *Ae. aegypti* can also transmit yellow fever. The US Gulf Coast region is therefore considered highly vulnerable to these arboviral infections [38], in addition to many of the other NTDs highlighted above. In a 2014 paper *in PLOS NTDs*, I identified the Gulf Coast as America's soft "underbelly" of NTDs [39]. Dr. Kristy O. Murray from our National School of Tropical Medicine recently determined that Houston is the first major US city to experience dengue fever epidemics in decades [40], and there are concerns that chikungunya or Zika arboviral infections will follow. In collaboration with Dr. Melissa Nolan Garcia, Murray's group has also found widespread West Nile virus (WNV) infections in Texas, where they cause serious neurologic and chronic renal disease [41–45]. More than three million WNV infections are estimated to have occurred over the past 15 years in the United States, and there are concerns that climate change may facilitate spread in the future [46]. Homeless populations are especially vulnerable to WNV infection [47].

The NTDs in the United States include toxocariasis, toxoplasmosis, trichomoniasis, cysticercosis, Chagas disease, and arboviral infections. Some of these diseases also have potent and serious effects on human mental health.

Given the panic and fear I saw over a single Ebola virus infection coming to Dallas in 2014, I am especially worried about the consequences of dengue, chikungunya, and Zika arboviral infections becoming widespread on the US Gulf Coast. These diseases can be extremely painful, and dengue is a significant cause of mortality, while Zika virus has been linked to microcephaly and other birth defects in Latin America. Accordingly, we are now working with both the Harris County and City of Houston health departments to shape a policy for communications and management if and when these arboviral infections emerge in our region.

HIV/AIDS and tuberculosis. According to the CDC, African Americans represent the racial/ethnic group most affected by HIV/AIDS, with a rate of new infection that is eight times that of whites [48]. Black men who have sex with men are disproportionately affected, often because of coinfections with other sexually transmitted diseases, as well as underdiagnosis, lack of access to care and treatment services, and decreased use of antiretroviral therapies [49]. African American women also suffer from high rates of infection [50]. Similarly, tuberculosis (TB) displays great health disparities, with 84% of the cases reported

HIV/AIDS and TB are diseases that reveal important health disparities in the United States.

among racial and ethnic minorities, including African Americans [51, 52]. However, the highest rates of TB infection are found in America's Pacific territories, led by the Marshall Islands, Micronesia, Guam, the Mariana Islands, and American Samoa, although Alaska and Hawaii also exhibit very high TB rates, as do the District of Columbia, California, and Texas [51, 52]. In terms of specific populations, the homeless and those incarcerated in correctional facilities exhibit especially high TB rates in the United States [51–53].

Raising Awareness

While interviewing on MSNBC, Fox News, and Bloomberg TV during the fall of 2014 at the height of West Africa's Ebola epidemic, which coincided with three Ebola cases in Dallas, I was sometimes questioned by anchors about my worries that Ebola virus infection would gain a foothold in the United States. I pointed out the unlikelihood that Ebola could take off in Texas or the rest of the nation, based on the difficulty of transmitting the virus in communities. Briefly, the viral loads associated with Ebola virus infection occur mostly among very sick and dying patients who are generally not mobile or moving about. Instead it is health-care workers and those tending to the sick and dying (or those burying the dead) who are at greatest risk of acquiring Ebola. Therefore, in the absence of a completely depleted health system, as we saw in Guinea, Liberia, and Sierra Leone, it is highly unlikely that Ebola virus infection could gain a foothold in the United States. However, while on national TV, I tried to use the opportunity to point out that although Americans were not at risk for Ebola virus infection, we already had 12 million Americans, mostly people living in poverty and people of color, living with at least one NTD. More often than not, the response from the TV anchor was generally, "Well, thank you doctor, but we're out of time."

NTDs in America have become an "inconvenient truth."

It has become apparent to me that NTDs in the United States represent an inconvenient truth. Many Americans have a difficult time admitting that we have 20 million fellow citizens who live at one-half the poverty level, perhaps 5 million who live on less than $2 per day, and 12 million who live with an NTD. It is ironic that educated people in the United States know far more about HIV/AIDS, TB, malaria, and even some NTDs in Africa and

Because tropical medicine is largely not taught in US medical schools, there is an extremely low awareness among US physicians and health-care providers about how to diagnose, manage, and treat NTDs.

India than they know about American NTDs. Even American physicians and other health-care providers know very little about the NTDs. Studies conducted by Dr. Susan Montgomery and her colleagues at the CDC in 2010 revealed that they knew next to nothing about Chagas disease, especially obstetricians, who are mostly unaware of the problem of mother-to-child transmission and congenital Chagas disease [54, 55]. Dr. Kristy Murray of our National School of Tropical Medicine tells me that none of the dengue patients identified in the 2003–5 epidemics in Houston was actually diagnosed by a physician!

The subjects of tropical medicine and parasitology are mostly not taught or barely mentioned in American medical schools and schools of nursing or allied health. In an effort to redress this problem, we have established a unique Diploma in Tropical Medicine at our National School of Tropical Medicine, run and organized by Dr. Laila Woc-Colburn, who also leads our tropical medicine clinic in collaboration with the Harris (County) Health System that provides much of the indigent care for greater Houston. Dr. Kathryn Jones runs our unique teaching laboratory for these diseases.

NTDs in the United States slip through the cracks.

Ultimately, NTDs in the United States slip through the cracks. Global health organizations such as the Bill & Melinda Gates Foundation do not recognize them because they are considered domestic rather than global health disparities, while simultaneously (and consistent with their eponymous neglected status) these NTDs have not been prioritized by the US Public Health Service or other branches of the US government.

Shaping a Policy and a Research and Development Agenda

The CDC has implemented policies for TB and HIV/AIDS among vulnerable and minority populations, but there is a need to also shape and develop similar policies for NTDs. At the state level, in collaboration with the Immunization Partnership—a local nongovernmental organization headed by Anna Dragsbaek, JD, and the Baylor College of Medicine—we worked with the legislature in Austin to introduce a bill for NTD surveillance in Texas. Texas

House Bill 2055, introduced by State Representative Sarah Davis of Houston (District 134) and State Senator Dr. Charles Schwertner (District 5), is the first to call for enhanced surveillance of NTDs [56]. But we need to expand surveillance for all the major NTDs across the United States. Led by US Representatives Hank Johnson (D-Georgia), Chris Smith (R-New Jersey), and others, the Neglected Infections of Impoverished Americans Act of 2015 (H.R. 2897) was reintroduced in the House of Representatives "to require the submission of a report to Congress on parasitic disease among poor Americans . . . with information necessary to address the threat posed by these diseases, evaluate current knowledge and gaps and guide future health policies" [57]. In parallel, US Rep. Chris Smith has sponsored an End Neglected Tropical Disease Act (H.R. 1797) [58], and US Rep. Gene Green, a Texas Democrat, has been leading efforts to introduce language about NTDs in the United States into the comprehensive 21st Century Cures Act [59]. I have been making frequent trips from Houston to Washington in order to keep American NTDs on the radar screen of US legislators, and I hope that some of these visits are now bearing fruit. In addition to surveillance, for some NTDs that are transmitted congenitally, such as Chagas disease and toxoplasmosis, we also need to expand efforts to test newborns, just as we currently conduct testing for genetic conditions such as phenylketonuria (table 10.4).

New NTD legislation has been passed in Texas, but it is pending in the US Congress.

We also need to better understand how these NTDs are actually transmitted within US borders, and I think it is extremely important to learn more about the links between these diseases and poverty. As I noted earlier, a drive through Houston's Fifth Ward provides some insights, as one can quickly identify predisposing risk factors, including stray animals, dilapidated houses without window screens, standing water and discarded tires, and other evidence of environmental degradation, but we need to conduct careful epidemiological studies to really understand the links between poverty and NTDs, as well as animal reservoirs for illnesses such as Chagas disease and others.

The major pillars of a policy that addresses American NTDs include (1) enhanced surveillance, (2) transmission studies, (3) prevention, and (4) new "control tools"—point-of-care diagnostics, drugs, and vaccines.

All of this presents an important research and development agenda for the NTDs in the United States. There are no point-of-care diagnostic tests available for most of the NTDs endemic to the nation, so blood from pa-

Table 10.4. Priority needs for enhanced surveillance, treatment, and prevention efforts for the high-priority neglected infections of poverty

Disease category	Disease	Expanded active surveillance and treatment	Newborn screening and treatment	Epidemiological transmission studies	New diagnostics	New drugs	New vaccines
Helminth infections	Ascariasis	+		+			+
	Toxocariasis	+		+	+		
	Strongyloidiasis	+		+	+		
	Cysticercosis	+		+	+	+	
Protozoan infections	Giardiasis	+					
	Cryptosporidiosis	+		+		+	
	Trichomoniasis	+					
	Chagas disease	+	+	+	+	+	+
	Leishmaniasis	+		+	+	+	+
	Congenital toxoplasmosis	+	+	+	+	+	+
Bacterial infections	Congenital syphilis		+	+			
	Brucellosis	+		+			
	Bovine tuberculosis	+		+			
	Trench fever	+		+			
	Leptospirosis	+		+			
Viral infections	Dengue fever	+		+		+	+
	Congenital cytomegalovirus	+	+	+		+	+

Source: [8], modified to include new information on leishmaniasis and Chagas disease vaccines, doi:10.1371/journal.pntd.0000256.t003.

tients must be sent to the CDC or other specialty research laboratories in order to establish a diagnosis for these conditions. As I sometimes point out to general audiences, when you go to your physician and get blood work done, there is no box to check off for toxocariasis or Chagas disease as there is for blood chemistries or other routine tests. We need diagnostic tests that are easily accessible to physicians and nurses.

We also need new and improved treatments and vaccines. Because the NTDs are poverty-related diseases, they often fly below the radar screen of the major pharmaceutical companies and are not prioritized. Thus, the drugs used to treat these illnesses are not widely available, so typically the CDC has to be contacted in order to access them. In addition, many of these medicines were developed decades ago and produce a lot of side effects. For instance, the two medicines for Chagas disease—benznidazole and nifurtimox—cause skin rashes, diarrhea, and other unpleasant or even dangerous symptoms and illnesses. Patients using these medications have to interrupt their treatments up to 20% of the time. Moreover, these drugs cannot be used by pregnant women.

So far the multinational pharmaceutical companies have shown little or modest interest in American NTDs. As a result, new products are being developed in the nonprofit sector.

Currently, new innovations for NTDs like Chagas disease still rely on nonprofit PDPs. The Geneva-based Drugs for Neglected Diseases Initiative is leading efforts to develop new and safer Chagas disease medicines [60], while at our National School of Tropical Medicine the Sabin Vaccine Institute and Texas Children's Hospital Center for Vaccine Development (Sabin PDP) is working to develop a therapeutic vaccine that could be used alongside existing treatments [61]. These efforts rely on major philanthropic donors. In our case at the Sabin PDP, they include the Kleberg Foundation, the Carlos Slim Foundation, the Southwest Electronic Energy Medical Research Institute, and Texas Children's Hospital.

Summary Points

1. In the United States, 45.3 million people live below the poverty line, roughly the same number of impoverished Americans alive during the early 1960s when Michael Harrington wrote *The Other America*. Approximately 20 million Americans now live in extreme poverty at

    one-half the US poverty level, and approximately 5 million are living on less than $2 per day.

2. American poverty concentrates in specific areas, especially in southern states, with Texas having the largest numbers who live in poverty. Important areas in the South include the Gulf Coast, border areas with Mexico, the Mississippi Delta, and Appalachia.

3. Approximately 12 million Americans are infected with NTDs, led by toxocariasis and trichomoniasis—which disproportionately affect African Americans—and Chagas disease (American trypanosomiasis) and cysticercosis—which disproportionately affect people of Hispanic origin. Toxoplasmosis is another important NTD. Toxocariasis, cysticercosis, and toxocariasis exert important mental health effects on impoverished Americans. Many of these NTDs are transmitted within US borders (autochthonous infections).

4. Arboviral infections are also important NTDs, led by dengue fever in Gulf Coastal areas and West Nile virus infection. WNV can cause chronic, persistent viral infections linked to chronic neurologic and renal disease.

5. There is an urgent need to promote awareness about the NTDs, especially for physicians and other health-care providers.

6. New policies are needed to expand surveillance for the NTDs affecting the United States. New legislation has been adopted in Texas, while additional bills are being introduced in the US Congress. Epidemiological studies are also needed to better understand how these diseases are transmitted and how they are linked to extreme poverty in the American South and elsewhere.

7. There is an urgent need for new "control tools" for American NTDs, including point-of-care diagnostics, antiparasitic and antiviral drugs, and vaccines. Many of these products are being developed by nonprofit PDPs rather than pharmaceutical companies.

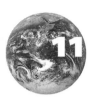

The G20

"A Theory of Justice"

In his landmark 1971 book *A Theory of Justice*, the Harvard political philosopher John Rawls articulates two overriding principles of a just and fair society, namely, (1) "equality in the assignment of basic rights and duties" and (2) allowance of some social and economic inequalities, but only if they ultimately benefit "the least advantaged members of society" [1]. In terms of Rawls's worldview, I believe that finding widespread NTDs among the extreme poor (and least-advantaged) who live amidst wealth—the central tenet of blue marble health—might represent one of the most jarring affronts to what he terms "justice as fairness."

Because NTDs are now widespread among the least-advantaged members of the world's wealthiest economies, and they represent a major basis for thwarting their future growth, it is urgent for these nations, especially the G20 countries, to adopt strong internal policies to combat these diseases. I envision a three-pronged strategy to best address the G20's (and Nigeria's) poorest citizens afflicted by NTDs:

> *Three major steps are required to effectively address blue marble health.*

1. Each of the G20 nations and Nigeria has the capacity to fully understand the extent of these diseases within their own borders and then provide their own impoverished populations access to essential medicines used in mass drug administration to target helminth infections, in addition to trachoma, leprosy, yaws and scabies, and to provide treatments for other high–disease burden NTDs, including leishmaniasis and Chagas disease. The G20 countries and Nigeria

need to allocate resources and implement programs to achieve universal coverage for these diseases.

2. Each of the G20 nations and Nigeria has the capacity to conduct research and development for new NTD biotechnologies; they need to allocate resources toward this goal.

3. Both activities should be conducted within an overall framework of health system strengthening.

Mass Drug Administration in the G20

A good place to revisit MDA among the G20 countries is to more closely examine the six G20 countries with positive worm indices—Brazil, China, India, Indonesia, Mexico, and South Africa—in addition to Nigeria. Together these countries account for one-half of the world's helminth infections [2]. An analysis of WHO's PCT database reveals that most of these nations are severely underachieving when it comes to providing MDA for people who require regular and periodic treatment for their intestinal helminth infections, schistosomiasis, and LF. Shown in table 11.1 is WHO's estimate of the percentage that received treatment in 2013 [3–5].

Overall, the G20 nations affected by helminth infections and Nigeria perform poorly when it comes to treating their affected populations through MDA. In terms of specific countries in Latin America, Brazil is reaching only approximately one-third of its children and population at risk. And although Mexico provides complete coverage for intestinal worms, it—as previously mentioned—neither diagnoses nor treats hundreds of thousands (and possibly millions) of people with Chagas disease. In Africa, Nigeria's MDA reaches less than 25% of its children at risk for helminth infections, and there is no information about schistosomiasis coverage in South Africa forthcoming from WHO. However, as Dr. Eyrun Kjetland (who works extensively in South Africa) has pointed out, female genital schistosomiasis remains widespread there, in part because praziquantel has been mostly unavailable in the country, owing to its drug importation laws. Schistosomiasis and other NTDs are still found among the poor in the Kingdom of Saudi Arabia. The entire MENA region severely underdiagnoses most of its NTDs, including leishmaniasis.

Table 11.1. WHO estimates of the percentage of people living in affected G20 countries and Nigeria who receive MDA

Country	% of school-age children at risk receiving deworming for their intestinal helminth infections in 2013 [3]	% of school-age children at risk receiving MDA for schistosomaisis in 2013 [4]	% of total population at risk receiving MDA for LF in 2013 [5]
Brazil	33.2 receiving albendazole	Not determined or available	27.5 receiving DEC
China	Not determined or available	Not determined or available	LF has been eliminated from China
India	15.7 receiving albendazole; 33.3 receiving albendazole + DEC	Schistosomiasis is not endemic to India	51.7 receiving DEC + albendazole
Indonesia	1.3 receiving albendazole; 7.6 receiving albendazole + DEC	55.8 receiving praziquantel (both children and adults)	24.5 receiving DEC + albendazole
Mexico	100 receiving albendazole	Schistosomiasis is not endemic to Mexico	LF is not endemic to Mexico
Nigeria	17.6 receiving albendazole + ivermectin 6.2 receiving albendazole + praziquantel	5.9 receiving praziquantel	19.7 receiving ivermectin + albendazole
South Africa	Not determined or available	Not determined or available	LF is not endemic to South Africa

Source: Table constructed from data in [3–5].

In Asia, Indonesia largely does not promote widespread deworming for its children, and only a small percentage of its population receives treatment for LF, while India does only marginally better. Indonesia also suffers from high rates of yaws, which can also be targeted by MDA using the antibiotic azithromycin. Similarly in India, the vast majority of its children do not have access to regular and periodic deworming, and only about one-half of the population receives MDA for LF. India also has the world's largest numbers of leprosy cases. This disease can also be attacked through MDA using a multidrug therapy regimen. WHO does not present information on China, either because it has not been determined or is unavailable. However, China has made great strides in reducing its schistosomiasis prevalence since 1949, and it has eliminated LF. Similarly, Japan and South Korea have achieved significant success both in economic development and in reducing or eliminating its NTDs.

Overall, the six G20 countries with positive worm indices, together with Nigeria, have the means and capacity to eliminate LF within their own borders, while greatly reducing the disease burdens of their intestinal helminth infections and schistosomiasis through MDA. Some of the key common factors for poor performance in meeting MDA targets are vast geographies, decentralization of health care that results in fragmentation of drug delivery, inadequate resource allocation, and lack of political will and commitment.

What about G20 countries affected by NTDs but without a positive worm index? In the United States, the 12 million Americans infected and living with NTDs are largely unrecognized, undiagnosed, and untreated. The United States also does very little in terms of conducting active surveillance for Chagas disease (and other major NTDs), and only a tiny percentage of its population receives access to diagnosis and treatment—the same is true for Argentina. In both North America and Europe, toxocariasis and other parasitic zoonotic infections are seldom diagnosed and treated. Minimal information is available on eastern Europeans, Turks, and Russians with intestinal worms or zoonotic NTDs or their access to diagnosis and treatment. NTDs remain widespread among Aboriginal Australians, including intestinal helminth infections and scabies—both of which can be targeted through MDA.

Thus, the current status of access to essential medicines for people living in poverty and with NTDs among the G20 countries and Nigeria can be summarized as abysmal. The fact that so few are being treated through MDA programs is especially sad, given its low costs. As previously mentioned, there are approximately 1.07 billion treatments required among the populations at greatest risk in the G20 countries and Nigeria. At a cost of 50 cents per person per year, approximately $500 million would be required—that is, a dollar amount representing a tiny percentage ($<0.001\%$) of the $65 trillion combined economy of these countries. The bottom line is that each of these nations has the internal capacity to provide these low-cost treatments to its impoverished populations.

WHO has now launched a Universal Health Coverage (UHC) initiative that builds on its 1978 "Health for All" Alma-Ata declaration and the Millennium Development Goals, with a focus on protecting the health of the world's most economically vulnerable populations. The activities highlighted here clearly fall within WHO's UHC mandate.

Research and Development for New Control Tools and Biotechnologies

For many of the leading NTDs—including vector-borne diseases such as dengue, leishmaniasis, Chagas disease, African sleeping sickness, and malaria, and also some helminth infections such as hookworm, schistosomiasis, onchocerciasis, and foodborne trematodiases—there are equally urgent needs to develop new drugs, diagnostics, and vaccines. Each year, the Australian policy group known as Policy Cures publishes an annual G-FINDER Report that measures the global investment in new technologies for neglected diseases, defining them broadly to include both the NTDs and the "big three" diseases: HIV/AIDS, TB, and malaria [6].

For the year 2014, G-FINDER determined that approximately $3.37 billion was invested globally in neglected disease R&D technology, with most of that support going toward the big three diseases [6]. A look at total government support for neglected disease R&D, almost all of it from G20 countries, is also interesting. The public sector provided 64% of the total funding, and the United States provided two-thirds of that funding, mostly from the US National Institutes of Health [6]. In all, 71% of the total government funding for neglected diseases comes from the United States, European Commission, and United Kingdom. However, as the G-FINDER Report points out, these absolute numbers do not consider the GDPs of these nations. In terms of public funding relative to GDP ratios, countries such as Ireland, Denmark, Norway, and Argentina do particularly well in this regard [6].

Shown in table 11.2 are selected estimates from G-FINDER of the percentage of their GDP that various governments have devoted to R&D on

Of government funding for neglected diseases R&D, a whopping 71% comes from the United States, European Commission, and United Kingdom. We need greater involvement and support from the remainder of the G20 countries, including positive worm index G20 countries— Brazil, China, India, Indonesia, Mexico, and South Africa, in addition to Nigeria.

neglected diseases. Using data from the G-FINDER Report combined with GDP information, I calculate that the world spends approximately 0.0028% of its GDP on neglected diseases R&D. Only three G20 countries—United States, United Kingdom, and Australia—match or exceed that percentage, although India and France come close to it. The worst-performing countries were China and Japan. However, in 2013 the Japanese government, together with Japan's major pharmaceutical companies and the Bill & Melinda Gates Foundation, formed a partnership known as the Global Health Innovative Technology (GHIT) Fund for supporting PDPs and other entities to develop and shape new biotechnologies for neglected diseases, with an emphasis on NTDs [7, 8]. China is a different matter. The *New York Times* has reported that China paid out $86.3 billion in foreign investments in the year 2013 [9], with much of that spent in fragile nations where health systems are broken and NTDs are widespread. Clearly, China needs to allocate some of those funds to neglected diseases, either for MDA or new technologies. In addition, the nation of Brazil could easily increase its global contribution to NTD technologies by 10-fold in order to match higher-performing nations in this regard.

Although NTDs and other poverty-related diseases account for almost 14% of the global disease burden, they receive only a bit more than 1% of the global health-related R&D funds.

Germany is now looking at supporting NTD technologies as part of an overarching G7 initiative on NTDs. In 2011, the German government launched a policy roadmap for neglected and poverty-related diseases [10]. Indeed, a recent analysis conducted by German investigators has found although NTDs and other poverty-related diseases account for almost 14% of the global disease burden, they receive only a bit more than 1% of the global health-related R&D funds [11].

R&D expenditures on helminth infections and neglected bacterial infections are ridiculously low.

As shown in figure 11.1, by presenting R&D expenditures for a particular disease divided by the disability adjusted life years (DALYs) it is possible to get a sense of diseases that are especially underfunded—even compared with other NTDS—such as the intestinal helminth infections and other neglected enteric diseases, as well as rheumatic fever [11]. Such data argue for the great urgency needed in addressing these health disparities by increasing R&D funding and support.

Table 11.2. Estimates of the percentage of GDP devoted by governments to R&D on neglected diseases

Country	GDP in 2014 (in trillions of US$)	R&D spending on neglected diseases in 2014 (in millions of US$)	% of GDP devoted to R&D on neglected diseases
European Union/European Commission	18.46	126	0.0007
United States	17.42	1,529	0.0087
China	10.36	< 11	<0.0001
Japan	4.60	11	0.0002
Germany	3.85	54	0.0014
United Kingdom	2.94	135	0.0046
France	2.83	73	0.0026
Brazil	2.35	11	0.0005
Italy	2.14	< 11	Not determined
India	2.07	40	0.0019
Russia	1.86	< 11	Not determined
Canada	1.79	17	0.0009
Australia	1.45	40	0.0028
South Korea	1.41	< 11	Not determined
Mexico	1.28	< 11	Not determined
Indonesia	0.89	< 11	Not determined
Turkey	0.80	< 11	Not determined
Saudi Arabia	0.75	< 11	Not determined
Nigeria	0.57	< 11	Not determined
Argentina	0.54	< 11	Not determined
South Africa	0.35	<11	Not determined
Global	77.89	2,165	0.0028

Source: R&D spending is either reproduced or calculated from information provided in [6]; 2014 GDP is from table 3.1.

Recently, the Dutch and German governments and the European Union (EU) have established important initiatives to support NTD R&D. The Dutch Ministry of Foreign Affairs, for instance, has been a major partner in our human hookworm vaccine initiative, while the EU has an important Frameworks Program 7 (FP7) for supporting new technologies [12], including a HOOKVAC Consortium of partners organized through the Amster-

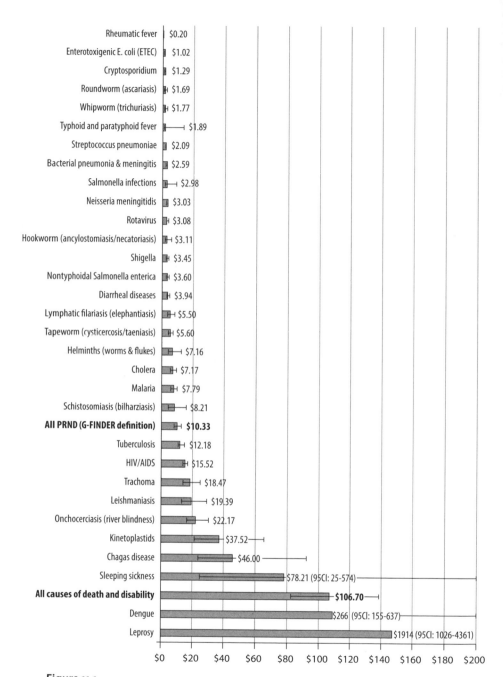

Figure 11.1.

Research and development expenditure (2008–12 annual average), by disease, in US dollars per DALY (2010). From [11].

dam Institute of Global Health and Development [13]. Most recently, the EU has established an ambitious Horizon 2020 program for expanding R&D in Europe, including NTD R&D activities [14], on top of a European and Developing Countries Clinical Trials Partnership (EDCTP) for clinically evaluating new NTD technologies [15]. New German government funding for NTD R&D funding was just announced. These Dutch, German, and EU initiatives represent an important advance for shaping the next generation of products to treat and prevent NTDs.

The US, Dutch, German, and Japanese governments, along with the EU, stand out for their contributions toward supporting product development to counter NTDs.

Yet another aspect of blue marble health is the rise in comorbid conditions between the NTDs, the big three diseases, and the noncommunicable diseases. Impoverished and neglected populations in the G20 countries and Nigeria are facing a double hit resulting from the convergence of NTDs and NCDs. For instance, in Texas, Mexico, and India (but presumably elsewhere) they include both TB and diabetes interactions and, lately, dengue and diabetes interactions. In South Africa, HIV/AIDS now flourishes amidst the high prevalence of female genital schistosomiasis. Studying the pathogenesis and epidemiology of these comorbid interactions will also be an important theme in the coming years.

Shaping a Policy for the G20

The G20 began meeting in 2008 in response to that year's global recession and have since convened in a summit each year to discuss the major policy issues of the day [16]. At the 2015 G20 Summit held in Turkey, the major areas of broad emphasis included strengthening the global recovery and enhancing resilience, while ensuring sustainability [17]. Clearly, lifting the bottom segments of their populations out of poverty through NTD control and elimination could fall within the G20 remit. It is imperative that the six member nations with positive worm indices commit to providing total MDA coverage for their populations affected by the major helminth infections, and also that the four Western Hemispheric countries step up surveillance, diagnosis, and treatment for Chagas disease. Leishmaniasis, both kala-azar and the cutaneous form, also represent major NTDs affecting the G20, and these diseases need to be targeted for control and elimination.

Equally important is the R&D agenda. There are some obvious under-achievers among the G20 countries that must step up and contribute to R&D for new drug, diagnostic, and vaccine products to fight the neglected diseases [18]. Toward that aim, several investigators have proposed the establishment of R&D funds to support neglected disease research. They include a global vaccine development fund [19] and a general biomedical R&D fund focused on antimicrobial resistance, emerging infectious diseases, and neglected diseases [20]. Both proposals are thoughtful, have a lot of merit, and need to be considered, but I offer an alternative or complementary solution. In 2013, the World Health Assembly passed a resolution (66.22) that proposes a "strategic work plan" to achieve sustainable funding for health R&D that could emphasize NTDs. The plan commits the director-general of the World Health Organization to establish a global "observatory" in order to identify gaps and opportunities for health R&D related to neglected diseases [21]. Through a pooled fund managed by WHO-TDR (a special program on tropical disease research and training), several pilot projects are now being supported [22].

Global funds for R&D are an option. An attractive alternative is to create national funds for product development R&D in each of the G20 countries and Nigeria—ones that resemble those put forward by the Dutch and Japanese governments.

Given that today's neglected disease R&D support comes mostly from the United States—and indeed mostly from a single agency, the National Institutes of Health—it is difficult to envision how such a fund would be created without calling on the NIH yet again. Realistically, it is unlikely the NIH leadership or the well-established community of US scientists would be willing to cede control of NIH budgets to an international body. Instead, I think it is worth considering the possibility of having each of the G20 countries establish its own version of the Japanese GHIT Fund, which builds on indigenous scientists and academic institutions and their own pharmaceutical industries. A Chinese or South Korean version of GHIT for example could become a vital and important institution. Creating twenty separate innovation funds could achieve the same goals as a global fund, while simultaneously ensuring national ownership and capacity building for indigenous academic and industrial institutions. Many of them could develop and shape new biotechnologies in collaboration with the 16 international PDPs. This approach would be especially useful for the less developed G20 countries, including Brazil,

India, Indonesia, and Mexico. These nations have indigenous vaccine manufacturers, which are represented by the Developing Country Vaccine Manufacturers Network, and therefore have a level of sophistication for producing next-generation NTD vaccines.

Still another option is for smaller groups of G20 countries to come together to support R&D investments. The EU's programs for new NTD technologies highlighted above represent important examples. In addition, if institutions from China and India (both rivals and neighbors) collaborated in the area of neglected diseases [23], some important NTD problems affecting Asia could be solved in the coming years. The United States has potential to extend its outreach on NTDs by collaborating with other G20 nations in the Americas or other countries [24].

As a UN agency, WHO could certainly partner with one or more of these G20 NTD R&D investment funds, especially through its global health R&D observatory mechanism. Another key United Nations agency might include WIPO—the World Intellectual Property Organization. Through the Patent Cooperation Treaty mechanism, the Geneva-based WIPO represents one of the few revenue-generating UN agencies. In 2011, in collaboration with BIO Ventures for Global Health, it established WIPO Re:Search to facilitate the development of products to combat NTDs by bringing together major pharmaceutical companies and academic investigators working on these diseases [25]. As a revenue-generating UN agency under the charismatic leadership of Francis Gurry, WIPO has the potential to expand this remit to support NTD product R&D.

Looking beyond the G20

The major NTDs linked to wealthy countries and blue marble health could also be addressed by nongovernmental organizations, including faith-based groups. For example, in 2011 the Pew Research Center's Forum on Religion and Public Life reported that the center of the world's Christian-majority countries has shifted from Europe and North America to the Global South, meaning Africa, Asia, and Central and South America [26]. Thus, countries such as Brazil, Philippines, Angola, Democratic Republic of Congo, and Papua New Guinea now have some of the highest percentages of Christian populations. As shown in table 11.3, from an analysis published in *PLOS NTDs*

Table 11.3. NTDs and global Christianity

Country or region (and rank)	Estimated 2010 Christian population (in millions)	Children requiring treatment for intestinal helminth infections in 2012 (in millions)	Population requiring treatment for schistosomiasis in 2012 (in millions)	Chagas disease cases (in millions)	Gambian human African sleeping sickness in 2012
Latin American and Caribbean (LAC) region (1)	533.9[a]	49.3	1.6	7.5	None
Philippines (2)	86.8	31.2	0.5	None	None
Nigeria (3)	80.5	65.4	60.6	None	2
China (4)	67.1	25.6	0.1	None	None
DR Congo (5)	63.1	29.2	18.0	None	5,983
Ethiopia (6)	52.6	32.3	22.1	None	None
South Africa (7)	40.6	3.2	5.2	None	None
Kenya (8)	34.3	16.7	11.8	None	None
Total	958.9	252.9	119.9	7.5	5,985
Global	7,200.0	875.9	249.4	7.8	7,106–7,216[b]
% in leading Christian countries	13%	29%	48%	96%	83–84%

Source: [26], doi:10.1371/journal.pntd.0003135.t001.
[a] Determined by subtracting the Christian populations of the United States (246.8 million) and Canada (23.4 million) from the total number of Christians living in the Americas (804.1 million).
[b] Two different numbers provided at http://www.who.int.

Most of the Christian-majority nations' populations now live in Africa, Asia, and Latin America. This finding opens up new possibilities of engagement with the Vatican and other types of governance linked to religion.

I found that almost all of the world's Chagas disease cases and African trypanosomiasis (sleeping sickness) can be found in Christian-majority countries, in addition to almost one-half of the schistosomiasis cases [26].

These findings suggest the possibility of bringing in new actors to combat NTDs. They could include the Vatican and Pope Francis, especially given the new pope's renewed commitment to impoverished populations [19]. The Orthodox Christian Church also has opportunities to highlight NTDs in countries such as Ethiopia or those in the Middle East, as do many Christian faith-based organizations and universities.

Summary Points

1. The six G20 countries with positive worm indices—Brazil, China, India, Indonesia, Mexico, and South Africa, together with Nigeria, have the means and capacity to eliminate LF within their own borders, while greatly reducing the disease burdens of their intestinal helminth infections and schistosomiasis through MDA.

2. G20 countries without classical worm indices, including the United States, also need to find mechanisms for promoting surveillance and access to essential medicine options for the poor living with NTDs within their own borders.

3. The G20 countries also have important biotechnology capabilities, which have yet to be adequately tapped for producing new NTD diagnostics, drugs, and vaccines. Beyond the United States, European nations, Australia, and Japan, they also include Brazil, China, India, Indonesia, Mexico, Russian Federation, Saudi Arabia, South Africa, and South Korea.

4. Yet another aspect of blue marble health is the rise in comorbid conditions between the NTDs, the big three diseases, and the NCDs.

5. The EU and the Dutch and German governments have launched important NTD technology initiatives, as has the Japanese government and its partners through a new GHIT Fund. These activities support PDPs committed to NTDs as well as indigenous academic institutions and industrial organizations.

6. Large G20 economies such as Brazil and China must increase their global commitment to support new NTD technologies and R&D.

7. There are opportunities to link these new investments with parallel activities ongoing at two UN agencies, namely, WHO and WIPO.

8. These topics should be highlighted at future G20 summits.

9. Faith-based organizations could have a future role. For instance, the Vatican and related entities have opportunities to expand commitments to control those NTDs that are found to be prevalent among Christian-majority countries.

12 A Framework for Science and Vaccine Diplomacy

entral to the blue marble health concept is that each of the G20 nations and Nigeria need to take greater responsibility for their own neglected diseases and neglected populations. Doing so could result in the control or elimination of one-half or more of the planet's NTDs, with substantial gains made against HIV/AIDS, TB, and malaria. Thus, while programs of overseas development assistance devoted to health, such as PEPFAR, GFATM, PMI, and USAID's NTD Program, in which the world's richest countries provide support to the poorest nations for their neglected diseases, must continue and should even expand, we need increasingly to recognize the hidden burden of neglected diseases among the poor living in wealthy countries.

As a first step, we must expand initiatives that raise awareness about the problem of NTDs within each of the G20 countries and Nigeria. The Global Network for NTDs linked to the Sabin Vaccine Institute has been working closely with the governments of India and Nigeria, respectively, in order to explain the opportunity for mass drug administration and its potential impact on health and economic development. MDA coverage rates are disappointingly low in these nations, especially for intestinal helminth infections and LF, as well as for schistosomiasis in the case of Nigeria. An extraordinary finding is that at least three nations with positive worm indices—India, Pakistan, and China—also maintain nuclear stockpiles [1]. Could the scientific horsepower of these nuclear states be partly redirected toward reducing endemic NTDs at home?

Outside of India and Nigeria, there is a need to promote NTD awareness in each of the G20 countries. For example, in the United States, our National School of Tropical Medicine has been highlighting the plight of some 12 million Americans living with NTDs. We have now worked with the Texas Legislature to enact a bill for NTD surveillance in suspected high-prevalence areas. However, similar initiatives need to be enacted across the G20 nations, including the European Union.

In addition, international cooperation between the different G20 nations and Nigeria could be critical in achieving higher population coverage for MDA. For instance, China, despite its billions of dollars of business investments in sub-Saharan Africa, has not yet promoted NTD control efforts there. Yet China has tremendous expertise in MDA for NTDs and could provide Africa with valuable advice in this area. China was the first country to eliminate LF and has achieved successes in reducing its burden of schistosomiasis more than 10-fold since the 1949 revolution. China could also share its best practices with neighboring India, where NTDs remain practically ubiquitous [2]. Similarly, Japan and South Korea have made great gains toward eliminating intestinal helminth infections, while the former has also successfully eliminated LF and schistosomiasis. International cooperation between these three East Asian nations and Nigeria, or with the G20 countries with positive worm indices, especially India, Indonesia, and Brazil (where they are the highest), could result in important, positive health and economic gains. Each of these activities represents examples of what some refer to as *global health diplomacy*.

Global health diplomacy initiatives between the G20 countries and Nigeria will be critical for achieving success in MDA programs and population coverage.

Global Health Diplomacy

My former colleague at Yale University, Ilona Kickbusch, currently the director of the Global Health Programme at the Graduate Institute of International and Development Studies in Geneva, has provided several working definitions of global health diplomacy, including efforts to "position health in foreign policy negotiations," together with the establishment of global health governance initiatives [3]. Indeed, the creation of the GAVI Alliance, GFATM, UNAIDS, and other Geneva-based organizations might

Major global health diplomacy initiatives launched since 2005 include IHR, GHSA, Global Health 2035, AAAA, and GFF.

be considered vital examples of organizations created under the auspices of global health diplomacy, with the first two created following the 2000 Millennial Development Goals. The MDGs themselves represent an important framework for global health diplomacy, and arguably the most successful.

Since 2005, several global health diplomacy initiatives have been enacted that could facilitate NTD activities among the G20 and Nigeria, although most of these actions are more focused on emerging viral infections of pandemic potential rather than the widespread chronic and debilitating NTDs.

- *The International Health Regulations (IHR)* were enacted in 2005 as a binding legal mechanism for all member states of WHO and focused on responses to acute public health emergencies [4]. IHR demands that countries report outbreaks and other public health events, while WHO responds with measures to uphold and enforce global health security [4]. IHR also establishes an emergency committee that advises the WHO director-general on whether an unexpected event should be considered a public health emergency. It also provides recommendations on initial steps for travel restrictions, surveillance, and infection control. With the possible exception of dengue fever, it is not clear how IHR will substantively address the NTDs or other blue marble health conditions. Moreover, even with IHR in place, the global response to the 2014 emergence of Ebola in West Africa was slow and inadequate and led to a catastrophic outbreak in the fall of that year [5]. This failure may require future revisions in the IHR, as recently recommended in a 2015 *Lancet* article by Lawrence Gostin and his colleagues at Georgetown University [6].
- *The Global Health Security Agenda (GHSA)* is an interagency initiative of the US government conducted in partnership with other nations and international organizations, including WHO [7]. GHSA is also focused on preventing or reducing the impact of epidemics and outbreaks of pandemic potential, such as H7N9 influenza virus or MERS coronavirus, as well as detecting emerging threats and imple-

menting rapid and effective responses. In some respects, GHSA represents the US component or response to IHR. It also covers intentional or accidental releases of dangerous infectious disease pathogens.

■ *Global Health 2035* and *The Lancet Commission* were launched in 2013, coinciding with the twentieth anniversary of a landmark 1993 World Development Report that helped to ignite international efforts to link investments in health with economic development [8]. The *Lancet* Commission identifies four key messages and actions: (1) the substantial economic return on investing in health, which can be as much as 24% in low- and middle-income countries; (2) implementation of a "grand convergence" in global health through scale-up of health technologies and strengthening health systems by the year 2035; (3) fiscal policies such as taxation of tobacco and reduction of subsidies for fossil fuels, which represent powerful forces or "levers" for elected leaders; and (4) universal health coverage as an efficient mechanism to improve health as well as to provide "financial protection" [8].

■ *The Addis Ababa Action Agenda (AAAA)* is the product of the first of three international meetings for implementing the UN's 2015 Sustainable Development Goals. However, health is at present only a minor component of the AAAA. Indeed, the SDGs have been criticized because health is now only 1 of the 17 goals, whereas it was front and center among the 2000 MDGs. So far, the AAAA's recommendations have included the promotion of the health systems strengthening component of the GFATM and GAVI Alliance and the establishment of a Global Financing Facility (GFF) for women's and children's health that would go hand-in-hand with the UN secretary general's new Global Strategy for Every Woman Every Child [9]. The emphasis of these initiatives is to reduce preventable maternal, child, and adolescent deaths by 2030. Despite the evidence that hookworm infection and Chagas disease rank among the leading complications of pregnancy among women living in poverty in low- and middle-income countries, while female genital schistosomiasis is among sub-Saharan Africa's most common gynecologic condition, there is not yet a specific mention of NTDs in the AAAA or GFF.

Ultimately, the G20 nations can identify ways to address blue marble health disparities under the auspices of the SDGs or the global health diplomacy initiatives highlighted above. However, at present there is no specific mandate for them to do so.

Vaccine Science Diplomacy

Concurrently, the G20 nations have opportunities to collaborate in scientific activities leading to the development of new drugs, diagnostics, and vaccines. I have used the term "vaccine science diplomacy" to refer to international scientific codevelopment of lifesaving vaccines between scientists of different nations, but particularly from nations with strained or evenly openly contentious international relations. The best historical example of vaccine science diplomacy is the codevelopment of the oral polio vaccine, led on the American side by Dr. Albert B. Sabin, and his Soviet virologist counterparts, including Dr. Mikhail Petrovich Chumakov [3].

Vaccine science diplomacy is a branch of science diplomacy that could lead to lifesaving vaccines developed between nations with strongly different ideologies.

In modern times there is potential interest in exploring vaccine science diplomacy opportunities between the United States and some of the world's Muslim-majority nations belonging to the Organisation of Islamic Cooperation [10, 11]. OIC countries include most of the Middle East and North Africa, as well as some highly populated Southeast Asian nations, including Bangladesh, Indonesia, and Malaysia, as well as most of central Asia.

New estimates that we published in *PLOS NTDs* in 2015 indicate that the 30 most-populated OIC countries account for 35% of the world's helminth infections comprising the global Worm Index, including 50% of the world's children who require MDA for schistosomiasis [11]. Given that approximately 1.5 billion people live in OIC countries, or about 20% of the global population, helminth infections appear to disproportionately affect the health and economic development of Muslim-majority countries, as does leishmaniasis, trachoma, and possibly other NTDs [11]. As shown in figure 12.1, there is also tight inverse association between the worm index and human development index in the Muslim world [11].

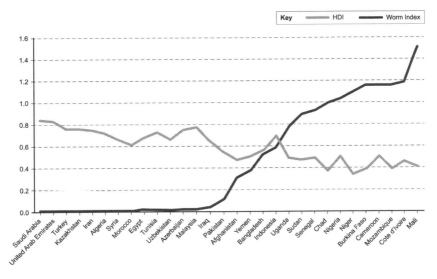

Figure 12.1.
Comparison of worm index versus the human
development index in the OIC countries. From [11].

OIC nations with strong infrastructures in science and biotechnology are potentially attractive candidates to pursue joint vaccine science diplomacy initiatives with the United States. Here the idea would be to promote scientific collaborations between US scientists and scientists from selected OIC countries in order to create new NTD technologies for some of the worst-off Muslim-majority countries. The "worst-off" might include OIC countries at the high end of the worm index, including Mali, Côte d'Ivoire, Mozambique, Cameroon, Burkina Faso, and Niger, as well as Nigeria [11].

The world's Muslim-majority OIC nations are disproportionately affected by NTDs and help to maintain a cycle of poverty in the Muslim world.

US Science Envoy Program

The beginnings of vaccine science diplomacy with OIC nations began in 2009, when the forty-fourth US president, Barack H. Obama, traveled to Cairo, where he delivered his landmark "New Beginnings" speech for reaching out to the Muslim world in the sciences, arts, and other areas [12, 13]. President Obama raised the following key points in his speech [13]:

> I've come here to Cairo to seek a new beginning between the United States and Muslims around the world, one based on mutual interest and mutual respect, and one based upon the truth that America and Islam are not exclusive and need not be in competition. Instead, they overlap, and share common principles—principles of justice and progress; tolerance and the dignity of all human beings.
>
> On science and technology, we will launch a new fund to support technological development in Muslim-majority countries, and to help transfer ideas to the marketplace so they can create more jobs. We'll open centers of scientific excellence in Africa, the Middle East and Southeast Asia, and appoint new science envoys to collaborate on programs that develop new sources of energy, create green jobs, digitize records, clean water, grow new crops. Today I'm announcing a new global effort with the Organization of the Islamic Conference to eradicate polio. And we will also expand partnerships with Muslim communities to promote child and maternal health.

A key action item following the president's trip was a subsequent announcement by then Secretary of State Hillary Clinton for establishing a US Science Envoy program, in which prominent US scientists—selected jointly by the White House Office of Science and Technology Policy and the US State Department—traveled to OIC nations in order to inaugurate joint collaborations. The initial cohort of US Science Envoys included former NIH director Elias Zerhouni, former National Academy of Sciences director Bruce Alberts, and Nobel laureate and professor from the California Institute of Technology Ahmed Zewail [12].

The US Science Envoy Program was launched to engage OIC countries in new initiatives in science diplomacy.

In December 2014, I was selected as a US science envoy, along with three other scientists who were committed to issues such as climate change and expanded opportunities for women in science. My activities focused on vaccine science diplomacy, with an emphasis on building capacity to develop vaccines in the MENA region. Since 2000, our Sabin Vaccine Institute PDP based at Texas Children's Hospital has led the development of new vaccines for diseases affecting the MENA and OIC countries, including schistosomiasis and other helminth infections, leishmaniasis, and MERS coronavirus infection [3, 14, 15]. Unlike most pharmaceutical companies or biotechs, our PDP is a nonprofit organization embedded in an academic health center, and it has the ability and experience to train and teach international scientists about the various steps in vaccine development, including antigen discovery, scale-up process development, manufacturing, regulatory filing, and phase 1 clinical testing [14, 15, 16].

In my role as US science envoy, I observed that there was a significant lack of connection between (1) the potential for dangerous NTDs and other neglected infectious diseases to emerge from Middle Eastern and North African (MENA) conflict zones, especially ISIS-occupied areas in Syria, Iraq, and Libya, as well as from Yemen, and (2) the ability of MENA scientific and industrial institutions to develop new vaccines for diseases emerging in the region. By and large, the big pharmaceutical companies and most biotechs are prepared to develop vaccines for global but not regional markets. Thus, without a new model and new interventions, vaccines for NTDs that mostly affect the MENA region might never be produced. Accordingly, I was invited to make visits to Morocco, Tunisia, and Saudi Arabia, based on their potential to expand or launch vaccine biotechnology initiatives, together with alignment of US foreign policy interests.

Both Tunisia and Morocco host Institut Pasteurs. These institutes have previously maintained capacity for developing some vaccines, such as BCG (TB vaccine) and rabies vaccines, which were first developed at the Institut Pasteur in Paris. The Tunisian Institut Pasteur still maintains that capacity. Moreover, the Kingdom of Saudi Arabia has sophisticated biotechnology infrastructures at several of its universities and research institutes, with capacity to build new-generation vaccines that require recombinant proteins or other genetic engineering methodologies. Geographically sandwiched between ISIS-occupied territories in Syria and Iraq to its north, and conflict in Yemen to its south, Saudi Arabia is especially vulnerable to the NTDs and emerging infections that could affect the MENA region [13–15]. In 2015, our Sabin Vaccine Institute signed a

There is an urgent need to build capacity in the MENA region for vaccine development. New vaccines will be needed to combat the NTDs emerging from the major conflict zones in Syria, Iraq, Libya, and Yemen. Through the US Science Envoy program, vaccine science diplomacy activities are under way to increase vaccine development capacity in selected MENA countries.

key agreement of cooperation with King Saud University's Prince Naif Bin Abdul Aziz Health Research Center for the purpose of creating a center of excellence for vaccine development. Areas of possible emphasis will include MERS coronavirus or leishmaniasis vaccines now urgently needed to combat those diseases in the MENA nations. Concurrently, we are also working with the University of Malaya to build vaccine development capacity in Southeast Asia. My hope is that the vaccines created through vaccine science diplomacy initiatives might become the first tangible deliverables of the blue marble health concept [16].

Summary Points

1. Central to the blue marble health concept is the realization that each of the G20 nations and Nigeria needs to accept greater responsibility for its own neglected diseases and neglected populations. Doing so could result in the control or elimination of one-half or more of the planet's NTDs, with substantial and similar gains in combating HIV/AIDS, TB, and malaria.

2. In parallel, international cooperation between the G20 countries and Nigeria could also promote NTD control and elimination initiatives. In particular three East Asian nations—China, Japan, and South Korea—each with a track record of success in NTD control, could work with Nigeria or with the G20 countries that have positive worm indices, especially India, Indonesia, and Brazil, where they are the highest. Such international cooperation could result in important, positive health and economic gains.

3. Today the GAVI Alliance, GFATM, and UNAIDS represent key Geneva-based global health cooperation and diplomacy organizations.

4. Since 2005, several new global health and health diplomacy initiatives have been launched, including IHR, GHSA, the *Lancet* Commission, AAAA, and GFF. However, it is unclear whether these initiatives are set up to adequately address the global NTD agenda.

5. In terms of new NTD drugs, diagnostics, and vaccines, there are opportunities to create science and vaccine diplomacy initiatives with the world's Muslim-majority OIC nations, which dispropor-

tionately account for the world's helminth infections, leishmaniasis, trachoma, and other NTDs.

6. OIC countries in the MENA region are now especially vulnerable to neglected and emerging infections arising from ISIS-occupied conflict zones in Syria, Iraq, and Libya, and from Yemen.

7. There is minimal capacity to develop vaccines in the MENA region. Through a US Science Envoy program, vaccine science diplomacy activities are under way to build vaccine development capacity in selected MENA countries.

8. The vaccines created through vaccine science diplomacy initiatives might become the first tangible deliverables of the blue marble health concept.

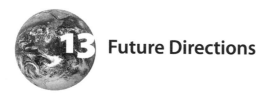 **Future Directions**

E ach of the major G20 nations and Nigeria is now contributing to the high global disease burden from the neglected tropical diseases, as well as HIV/AIDS, TB, malaria, and the noncommunicable diseases. With regard to the NTDs, these same nations must assume greater roles and responsibilities in leading control and elimination efforts. The G20 and Nigeria can effect major changes both within their borders and internationally. If fully realized, the global burden of the major NTDs can be reduced by one-half in the case of the helminth infections and by two-thirds or more for some of the other vector-borne NTDs and leprosy. According to the Global Burden of Disease Study 2013, the 17 major NTDs and malaria together accounted for 20.1 million years lived with disability (YLDs) and 997,000 deaths [1, 2], so by addressing these blue marble health issues, the G20 nations and Nigeria could prevent millions of years lived with disability and hundreds of thousands of deaths. Yet another aspect of blue marble health is the rise in comorbid conditions between the NTDs, the big three diseases, and the NCDs.

The specific suggestions for creating a blue marble health framework have been detailed throughout this book. Some of the major policy and other recommendations include steps to promote mass drug administration within national borders and to expand research and development efforts to create new drugs, diagnostics, and vaccines, while pursuing overall goals directed at strengthening health systems.

China. China has been a trendsetter and pioneer in the battle against NTDs, having been the first large nation to eliminate LF through MDA and having made great strides since its 1949 revolution in nearly eliminating schistosomiasis from the Yangtze River valley. China now needs to expand these efforts to control intestinal helminth infections in its southwestern region and malaria near the Burma border, and then to begin chipping away at a worrisome problem with liver and lung fluke infections. Simultaneously, China can do much more to export its expertise and experience in parasite and NTD control, especially to Africa, where it currently invests billions of dollars in the extraction of minerals and fossil fuels. China also has tremendous but underused capacity for innovation. China may be the world's largest producer of vaccines, and like India is now exporting low-cost affordable vaccines [3]. But it needs to do more to develop new NTD vaccines beyond its success with a vaccine for Japanese encephalitis. Also on the R&D front, China has to commit resources to establish a well-financed global health innovation technology fund similar to Japan's GHIT initiative. Such a fund would be transformative.

Japan and South Korea. These two Asian nations also have a great post–World War II history of eliminating their NTDs (although aided in part by aggressive economic development and urbanization during that era), and like China could offer advice and expertise on MDA and health system strengthening to impoverished areas of Africa and Asia. Japan has now established a successful GHIT Fund to spur NTD innovations in partnership with its industrial and academic institutions; South Korea can do the same.

Indonesia and India. MDA for Indonesia's major NTDs, including LF, intestinal helminth infections, and yaws, faces logistical challenges because of the nation's vast and complicated island geography. In addition, Indonesia has decentralized its health-care system, leading to fragmentation of drug delivery, and the political will required to confront its internal NTD problem remains in question. Indonesia has the ability to develop vaccines, and this skill needs to be better exploited in the service of innovative treatment and control measures to counter NTDs. Similar political and social factors have previously been responsible for inconsistent or inadequate delivery of MDA in India. Malaria has emerged as a major killer in India and South Asia. However, India is becoming more ambitious in tackling LF, as MDA drug coverage now exceeds the 50% mark, and the government has also created National Deworming Days for intestinal helminth infections in children and adolescents. These national efforts represent good starts, but India must continue on this trajectory, while also redoubling efforts to implement case detection and treatment for kala-azar and, if possible, scaling up indigenous production of liposomal amphotericin B. India could also play a greater role in ensuring that its South Asian neighbors increase their NTD interventions. Like China, India has enormous pharmaceutical and vaccine development capacity, and it is beginning to have some important successes in producing new, groundbreaking NTD products. Some of these innovations are being catalyzed through collaborations with nonprofit PDPs. The key to innovation for NTDs globally partly rests on the shoulders of India.

Both Indonesia and India are reeling under massive dengue fever epidemics. Aside from the public health burden caused by dengue and its medical complications are the huge health-care costs and lost economic productivity associated with this disease. In addition to the requirement for intensified vector control and management, the vaccine development capabilities of India and Indonesia have great potential for leadership in new dengue vaccines.

Nigeria. Today, Nigeria has the largest number of people in Africa living with NTDs. However, the nation also has the internal resources and the economy to massively expand its current government commitment for indigenous NTD control and elimination efforts through MDA, especially for LF, onchocerciasis, intestinal helminth infections, and schistosomiasis. The forces that thwart MDA for NTDs in Nigeria are similar to those in Indonesia and India: complicated logistics, decentralization and fragmented delivery of essential medicines, inadequate allocation of resources, and insufficient political will. In the case of Nigeria, the presence of Boko Haram has further hampered MDA efforts in the north. If they were better financially supported, Nigeria's research institute and universities could also assume a greater role in spurring innovation nationally and for Africa.

South Africa. South Africa has one of the worst HIV/AIDS epidemics in the world. While the South African government has done much to provide access to essential medicines for antiretroviral therapy, it mostly ignores one of its major AIDS cofactors in KwaZulu-Natal, namely, co-endemic female genital schistosomiasis. This situation must change through increased MDA with praziquantel. South Africa also has some important R&D infrastructure that can be further tapped for the development of NTD control products.

Saudi Arabia and the MENA region. Saudi Arabia and other nations of the MENA region face a new threat from NTDs emerging out of conflict zones and the associated breakdowns in health systems in ISIS-occupied Syria, Iraq, and Libya, as well as Yemen. The diseases include leishmaniasis,

MERS coronavirus infection, and arboviral infections. Additional threats in Saudi Arabia include hidden poverty and diseases introduced annually from OIC countries in Africa and Asia during the Hajj, the annual pilgrimage to Mecca. Overall, given its oil and energy wealth and the high quality of some of its research universities and institutes, the MENA region overall has underachieved in terms of its ability to make new products, especially vaccines. Of particular concern are products for its diseases of regional, but not necessarily global, importance. These illnesses fall through the cracks because they are of less interest to multinational pharmaceutical companies. Now, through the US Science Envoy program, scientific collaborations are expanding with PDPs, including our Sabin Vaccine Institute and Texas Children's Hospital Center for Vaccine Development. Together, a Saudi Arabian–PDP alliance could foster a new generation of antipoverty interventions for NTDs in the OIC nations.

Argentina, Brazil, and Mexico. In northern Argentina, northeastern Brazil, and southern Mexico, NTDs remain widespread. In Argentina and Brazil, MDA for intestinal helminth infections needs to expand, as does MDA for schistosomiasis in Brazil. Brazil has the capacity to eliminate both LF and schistosomiasis, each historically introduced through the Atlantic slave trade. Arboviruses represent important threats to the economies of all three nations, and for me it is a disappointment that innovation in the way of new vaccines to combat dengue have so far not emerged from any of these countries. Now Zika and chikungunya further threaten the Latin American region.

Most of the world's Chagas disease cases are found in Argentina, Brazil, and Mexico, representing the three wealthiest nations in Latin America. Sadly, less than 1% of the individuals living with Chagas disease receive access to diagnosis and treatment. Chagas disease is truly a forgotten disease among forgotten people living alongside Latin America's wealthy elite, and an important disease in terms of preserving the region's notoriously high GINI indexes. Together, Argentina, Brazil, and Mexico can also provide leadership for NTD prevention and treatment measures in the poorest nations in the Americas, including Central American countries and Bolivia, where the prevalence of these illnesses is the highest. The capacity for innovation is high in Latin America—especially for Brazil, which is now working to develop new dengue vaccines—but also in nations such as Argentina, Mexico, and Cuba. Some of these activities are being conducted in collaboration with PDPs.

Australia and Canada. The aboriginal peoples of Australia and Canada suffer high rates of unique NTDs. In Australia, the major NTDs such as intestinal helminth infections, trachoma, and scabies could potentially be eliminated through stepped-up MDA efforts. In Canada, the major NTDs are foodborne zoonotic parasitic infections affecting the Arctic region, but there is a threat of emerging arboviral infections resulting from climate change. The Australian and Canadian governments have both made commitments to addressing these health disparities, but their depth and breadth are unclear.

European Union, Russian Federation, and Turkey. In Europe, the Russian Federation, and Turkey, the major NTDs include parasitic zoonoses, but there is also now a serious threat from vector-borne diseases, especially arboviral infections and vivax malaria, in southern Europe. Diseases arising out of the ISIS-conflict zones also pose a risk to Turkey, southern Europe, and Russia. Climate change is another important consideration and factor. German-led efforts through the G7 are looking at how MDA efforts can be enhanced worldwide, while currently the UKAID and the British DFID are the largest supporters of MDA aside from USAID. Through its Frameworks and Horizon 2020 programs, the European Union is working hard to finance and stimulate innovations to combat NTDs. Additional and highly welcomed initiatives are coming from the Dutch, UK, and German governments, among others.

United States. In the United States, an estimated 12 million people live with an NTD, especially in Texas, the Gulf Coast, and the South. The major NTDs include five neglected parasitic infections—Chagas disease, cysticercosis, toxocariasis, toxoplasmosis, and trichomoniasis—in addition to emerging arboviral infections, including dengue and West Nile virus infection. There is virtually no surveillance activity for NTDs in the United States, so most of these diseases go undiagnosed, but new legislation recently passed in Texas and currently under consideration by the US Congress could change this situation. There are also urgent needs to better understand how these American NTDs are transmitted within US borders and to develop new and improved point-of-care diagnostics, as well as drugs and vaccines. Most physicians and health-care providers are largely unaware of the public health threat of American NTDs, a gap we are trying to close at our National School of Tropical Medicine at Baylor College of Medicine. In terms of supporting scientific efforts to treat and control NTDs, the

National Institutes of Health is by far the leading government funder of neglected diseases R&D, but much of this activity is focused on basic research. More US government support is needed for translational and product development, as well as for PDPs [4]. Through its USAID Program, the US government is also the largest donor for MDA.

Global partnerships. Much of the global governance for NTD control and elimination falls on the World Health Organization. Approximately 40% of the world's population that requires MDA now receives access to essential NTD medicines through WHO, working in collaboration with a consortium of partners, including ministries of health and their community-based drug distributors and some key nongovernmental organizations [5]. Falling into the big gaps in treatment coverage among the other 60% are the vulnerable populations living in the G20 countries and Nigeria. The annual G20 summits and the preparatory meetings leading up to them provide a potential new venue for ensuring that these neglected populations have access to NTD medicines. But beyond mass drug administration, there is an urgent need to create new products. There is a significant level of innovation among selected countries of the G20, especially in large middle-income countries such as Argentina, Brazil, China, India, Indonesia, and Mexico, as well as in Saudi Arabia, where member organizations of the Developing Country Vaccine Manufacturers Network operate [6]. These efforts are partly monitored through WHO's new Product Development for New Vaccines Advisory Committee and the Special Programme for Research and Training in Tropical Diseases, but again the G20 government leaders need to assume a greater role in spurring medical advances in the prevention and treatment of those diseases that disproportionately afflict the most vulnerable populations in their countries [7]. People living in poverty not only have a fundamental human right of access to essential medicines, but to innovation as well. An attractive mechanism for each nation might resemble what Japan has done through its GHIT Fund, such that each of the G20 countries could create a similar mechanism but with its own unique national character. Global funds for innovation also offer promise, but these multinational mechanisms bring with them added complexities. One new auspicious approach is through the World Intellectual Property Organization, whose Re:-Search organization has created some links between academic partners and industry. I believe that WIPO, as a self-supporting UN agency through its revenue-generating supervision of patents under the Patent Cooperation

Treaty, could further tap into this mechanism to spawn funds for product development partnerships committed to NTDs.

The concept of blue marble health helps to illustrate some key failings among the elected leaders and the leadership of the G20 countries in looking after the weakest members of their nations. Today, hundreds of millions of people living in the G20 are essentially ignored and lack access to essential medicines, innovation, or health systems. As Elie Wiesel once said, "The opposite of love is not hate; it's indifference."

Literature Cited

Introduction

1. Hotez PJ (2013) The disease next door. Foreign Policy, March 25.
2. Hotez PJ (2013) NTDs V.2.0: "Blue marble health"—Neglected tropical disease control and elimination in a shifting health policy landscape. PLOS Negl Trop Dis 7: e2570.
3. Petsko GA (2011) The blue marble. Genome Biol 12: 112.

Chapter 1. A Changing Landscape in Global Health

1. Hotez PJ (2013) Forgotten people, forgotten diseases: The neglected tropical diseases and their impact on global health and development. Washington, DC: ASM Press.
2. Hotez PJ, Bottazzi ME, Strych U (2016) New vaccines for the world's poorest people. Annu Rev Med, in press.
3. GBD 2013 Mortality and Causes of Death Collaborators (2015) Global, regional, and national age-sex specific all-cause and cause-specific mortality for 240 causes of death, 1990–2013: A systematic analysis for the Global Burden of Disease Study 2013. Lancet 385: 117–71.
4. Larson HJ, Schulz WS, Tucker JD, Smith DMD (2015) Measuring vaccine confidence: Introducing a global vaccine confidence index. PLOS Currents Outbreaks, February 25, edition 1; doi: 10.1371/currents.outbreaks.ceof6177bc97332602 a8e3fe7d7f7cc4.
5. Hotez P (2015) "Vaccine hesitancy": The PLOS Currents collection. PLOS Speaking of Medicine blog, February 25, http://blogs.plos.org/speakingofmedicine /2015/02/25/vaccine-hesitancy-plos-currents-collection.
6. Hotez PJ (2015) Protecting kids: My experience with vaccine refusal and autism awareness. PATH #ProtectingKids blog series, http://www.sabin.org

/updates/blog/protecting-kids-my-experience-vaccine-refusal-and-autism
-awareness.

7. Stoner R, Chow ML, Boyle MP, Sunkin SM, Mouton PR, Roy S, Wynshaw-
Boris A, Colamarino SA, Lein ES, Courchesne E (2014) Patches of disorganization
in the neocortex of children with autism. N Engl J Med 370(13): 1209–19.

8. Hotez PJ (2014) Blue marble health: A new presidential roadmap for global
poverty-related diseases. James A. Baker III Institute for Public Policy, Rice University, http://bakerinstitute.org/research/blue-marble-health-new-presidential
-roadmap-global-poverty-related-diseases.

9. Murray CJL, Ortblad KF, Guinovart C, Lim S, Wolock TM, et al. (2014)
Global, regional, and national incidence and mortality for HIV, tuberculosis, and
malaria during 1990–2013: A systematic analysis for the Global Burden of Disease
Study 2013. Lancet 384: 1005–70.

10. Murray CJL, Vos T, Lozano R, Naghavi M, Flaxman AD, et al. (2012)
Disability-adjusted life years (DALYs) for 291 diseases and injuries in 21 regions,
1990–2010: A systematic analysis for the Global Burden of Disease Study 2010.
Lancet 380: 2197–223.

11. Jamison DT, Summers LH, Alleyne G, Arrow KJ, Berkley S, et al. (2013)
Global health 2035: A world converging with a generation. Lancet 382: 1898–955.

12. Hotez PJ, Daar AS (2008) The CNCDs and the NTDs: Blurring the Lines
Dividing Noncommunicable and Communicable Chronic Diseases. PLoS Negl
Trop Dis 2(10): e312; doi:10.1371/journal.pntd.0000312.

Chapter 2. The "Other Diseases"

1. http://www.who.int/nmh/events/2014/high-level-unga/en.

2. Jamison DT, Summers LH, Alleyne G, Arrow KJ, Berkley S, et al. (2013)
Global health 2035: A world converging with a generation. Lancet 382: 1898–955.

3. Hotez PJ (2013) Forgotten people, forgotten diseases: The neglected tropical
diseases and their impact on global health and development. Washington, DC:
ASM Press.

4. http://www.ibtimes.com/how-three-scientists-marketed-neglected-tropical
-diseases-raised-more-1-billion-1921008.

5. Molyneux DH, Hotez PJ, Fenwick A (2005) "Rapid-impact interventions":
How a policy of integrated control for Africa's neglected tropical diseases could
benefit the poor. PLOS Med 2(11): e336; doi:10.1371/journal.pmed.0020336.

6. Hotez PJ, Molyneux DH, Fenwick A, Ottesen E, Ehrlich Sachs S, Sachs JD
(2006) Incorporating a rapid-impact package for neglected tropical diseases with
programs for HIV/AIDS, tuberculosis, and malaria. PLOS Med 3(5) (January):
e102.

7. Hotez PJ, Molyneux DH, Fenwick A, Kumaresan J, Sachs SE, Sachs JD, Savioli L (2007) Control of neglected tropical diseases. N Engl J Med. 357(10) (September 6): 1018–27.

8. GBD 2013 Disease and Injury Incidence and Prevalence Collaborators (2015) Global, regional, and national incidence, prevalence, and YLDs for 301 acute and chronic diseases and injuries for 188 countries, 1990–2013: A systematic analysis for the Global Burden of Disease Study 2013. Lancet 386(9995): 743–800.

9. Hampson K, Coudeville L, Lembo T, Sambo M, Kieffer A, Attlan M, et al. (2015) Estimating the global burden of endemic canine rabies. PLOS Negl Trop Dis 9(4): e0003709; doi:10.1371/journal.pntd.0003709.

10. Hotez PJ, Daar AS (2008) The CNCDs and the NTDs: Blurring the lines dividing noncommunicable and communicable chronic diseases. PLOS Negl Trop Dis 2(10): e312; doi:10.1371/journal.pntd.0000312.

11. Hotez PJ, Ferris MT (2006) The antipoverty vaccines. Vaccine 24(31–32) (July 26): 5787–99.

12. Hotez PJ, Fenwick A, Savioli L, Molyneux DH (2009) Rescuing the bottom billion through control of neglected tropical diseases. Lancet 373(9674) (May 2): 1570–75; doi: 10.1016/S0140-6736(09)60233-6.

13. Hotez P, Whitham M (2014) Helminth infections: A new global women's health agenda. Obstet Gynecol 123(1) (January): 155–60; doi: 10.1097/AOG.000000 0000000025.

14. Litt E, Baker MC, Molyneux D (2012) Neglected tropical diseases and mental health: A perspective on comorbidity. Trends Parasitol 28(5) (May): 195–201; doi: 10.1016/j.pt.2012.03.001.

15. Weiss MG (2008) Stigma and the social burden of neglected tropical diseases. PLOS Negl Trop Dis 2(5): e237; doi:10.1371/journal.pntd.0000237.

16. Hotez PJ, Herricks JR (2015) Helminth elimination in the pursuit of sustainable development goals: A "worm index" for human development. PLOS Negl Trop Dis 9(4): e0003618; doi:10.1371/journal.pntd.0003618.

17. https://sustainabledevelopment.un.org/focussdgs.html.

18. http://unitingtocombatntds.org/resource/london-declaration.

19. De Clercq D, Sacko M, Behnke J, Gilbert F, Dorny P, Vercruysse J (1997) Failure of mebendazole in treatment of human hookworm infections in the southern region of Mali. Am J Trop Med Hyg 57(1) (July): 25–30.

20. Albonico M, Bickle Q, Ramsan M, Montresor A, Savioli L, Taylor M (2003) Efficacy of mebendazole and levamisole alone or in combination against intestinal nematode infections after repeated targeted mebendazole treatment in Zanzibar. Bull World Health Organ 81(5): 343–52.

21. Soukhathammavong PA, Sayasone S, Phongluxa K, Xayaseng V, Utzinger J, Vounatsou P, Hatz C, Akkhavong K, Keiser J, Odermatt P (2012) Low efficacy of single-dose albendazole and mebendazole against hookworm and effect on concomitant helminth infection in Lao PDR. PLOS Negl Trop Dis 6(1) (January): e1417; doi: 10.1371/journal.pntd.0001417.

22. Keiser J, Utzinger J (2008) Efficacy of current drugs against soil-transmitted helminth infections: Systematic review and meta-analysis. JAMA 299(16) (April 23): 1937–48; doi: 10.1001/jama.299.16.1937.

23. Albonico M, Smith PG, Ercole E, Hall A, Chwaya HM, Alawi KS, Savioli L (1995) Rate of reinfection with intestinal nematodes after treatment of children with mebendazole or albendazole in a highly endemic area. Trans R Soc Trop Med Hyg 89(5) (September–October): 538–41.

24. http://www.neglecteddiseases.gov.

25. WHO (2015) Planning, requesting medicines and reporting for preventive chemotherapy. Weekly Epidemiol Rec 90(14): 133–48.

26. Keenan JD, Hotez PJ, Amza A, Stoller NE, Gaynor BD, Porco TC, et al. (2013) Elimination and eradication of neglected tropical diseases with mass drug administrations: A survey of experts. PLOS Negl Trop Dis 7(12): e2562; doi:10.1371 /journal.pntd.0002562.

27. Hotez PJ, Pecoul B, Rijal S, Boehme C, Aksoy S, Malecela M, Tapia-Conyer R, Reeder JC (2016) Eliminating the neglected tropical diseases: Translational science and new technologies. PLOS Negl Trop Dis 10(3): e0003895; doi:10.1371/ journal.pntd.0003895.

28. Hotez PJ, Beaumier CM, Gillespie PM, Strych U, Hayward T, Bottazzi ME (2016) Advancing a vaccine to prevent hookworm disease and anemia. Vaccine [Epub ahead of print: https://www.ncbi.nlm.nih.gov/pubmed/27040400].

29. Merrifield M, Hotez PJ, Beaumier CM, Gillespie P, Strych U, Hayward T, Bottazzi ME (2016) Advancing a vaccine to prevent human schistosomiasis. Vaccine [Epub ahead of print: https://www.ncbi.nlm.nih.gov/pubmed/27036511].

30. Lee BY, Bacon KM, Bailey R, Wiringa AE, Smith KJ (2011) The potential economic value of a hookworm vaccine. Vaccine 29(6): 1201–10.

Chapter 3. Introducing Blue Marble Health

1. Molyneux DH, Hotez PJ, Fenwick A (2005) "Rapid-impact interventions": How a policy of integrated control for Africa's neglected tropical diseases could benefit the poor. PLOS Med 2(11): e336; doi:10.1371/journal.pmed.0020336.

2. World Bank (1993) World Development Report, https://openknowledge .worldbank.org/handle/10986/5976.

3. Marmot M (2005) Social determinants of health inequalities. Lancet 365: 1099–104.

4. https://g20.org/about-g20.

5. Hotez PJ (2015) Blue marble health redux: Neglected tropical diseases and human development in the Group of 20 (G20) nations and Nigeria. PLOS Negl Trop Dis 9(7): e0003672.

6. http://databank.worldbank.org/data/download/GDP.pdf.

7. The World Bank. Data. European Union, http://data.worldbank.org/country /EUU, accessed February 2, 2015.

8. Worldometers. Population, http://worldometers.info/world-population/pop ulation-by-country, accessed February 11.

9. https://data.oecd.org/gdp/gross-domestic-product-gdp.htm.

10. Hotez PJ (2013) The disease next door. Foreign Policy, March 25.

11. Hotez PJ (2013) NTDs V.2.0: "Blue marble health"—Neglected tropical disease control and elimination in a shifting health policy landscape. PLOS Negl Trop Dis 7: e2570.

12. Petsko GA (2011) The blue marble. Genome Biol 12: 112.

13. Murray CJL, Vos T, Lozano R, Naghavi M, Flaxman AD, et al. (2012) Disability-adjusted life years (DALYs) for 291 diseases and injuries in 21 regions, 1990–2010: A systematic analysis for the Global Burden of Disease Study 2010. Lancet 380: 2197–223.

14. Global Burden of Disease Study 2013 Collaborators (2015) Global, regional, and national incidence, prevalence, and years lived with disability for 301 acute and chronic diseases and injuries in 188 countries, 1990-2013: a systematic analysis for the Global Burden of Disease Study 2013. Lancet 386: 743–800.

15. World Health Organization, Neglected Tropical Diseases, PCT Databank. Soil-transmitted helminthiases, http://www.who.int/neglected_diseases/preventive _chemotherapy/sth/en, accessed February 5, 2015.

16. World Health Organization (2014) Soil-transmitted helminthiases: Number of children treated in 2012. Weekly Epidemiol Rec 89(13): 133–40.

17. World Health Organization, Neglected Tropical Diseases, PCT Databank. Schistosomiasis, http://www.who.int/neglected_diseases/preventive_chemotherapy /sch/en, accessed February 5, 2015.

18. World Health Organization (2014) Schistosomiasis: Number of people receiving preventive chemotherapy in 2012. Weekly Epidemiol Rec 89(2): 21–28.

19. World Health Organization, Neglected Tropical Diseases, PCT Databank. Lymphatic filariasis, http://www.who.int/neglected_diseases/preventive_chemo therapy/lf/en.

20. World Health Organization (2014) Global programme to eliminate lymphatic filariasis: Progress report, 2013. Weekly Epidemiol Rec 89(38): 409–20.

21. World Health Organization (2014) African Programme for Onchocerciasis Control: Progress report, 2013–2014. Weekly Epidemiol Rec 89(49): 551–60.

22. Hotez PJ, Herricks JR (2015) Helminth elimination in the pursuit of sustainable development goals: A "worm index" for human development. PLOS Negl Trop Dis 9(4): e0003618.

23. Bhatt S, Gething PW, Brady OJ, Messina JP, et al. (2013) The global distribution and burden of dengue. Nature 496: 504–7.

24. World Health Organization (2014) Global leprosy update, 2013: Reducing disease burden. Weekly Epidemiol Rec 36(89): 389–400.

25. Hotez PJ (2014) Blue marble health: A new presidential roadmap for global poverty-related diseases. James A Baker III Institute for Public Policy, Rice University, http://bakerinstitute.org/research/blue-marble-health-new-presidential -roadmap-global-poverty-related-diseases.

26. https://www.iom.edu/Global/Perspectives/2013/StrengtheningMechanisms RD.aspx.

27. Hotez PJ (2015) Blue marble health and "the big three diseases": HIV/AIDS, tuberculosis, and malaria. Microbes Infec 17(8): 539–41.

28. From annex table 3: People living with HIV (all ages), 2005 and 2013, pp. A18–A23. In: UNAIDS. The Gap Report, http://www.unaids.org/en/resources/documents /2014/20140716_UNAIDS_gap_report.

29. Centers for Disease Control and Prevention, http://www.cdc.gov/hiv/statistics /basics/ataglance.html.

30. From table 2.1: Estimated epidemiological burden of TB, 2013, p. 13. In: World Health Organization. Global Tuberculosis Report 2014, http://www.who.int /tb/publications/global_report/en.

31. Centers for Disease Control and Prevention, National Center for HIV/AIDS, Viral Hepatitis, STD, and TB Prevention. Reported Tuberculosis in the United States 2013, http://www.cdc.gov/tb/statistics/reports/2013/pdf/report2013.pdf.

32. From annex 6A: Reported malaria cases and deaths, 2013, pp. 202–4. In: World Health Organization. World Malaria Report 2014, http://www.who.int /malaria/publications/world_malaria_report_2014/en.

33. Centers for Disease Control and Prevention, http://www.cdc.gov/malaria /about/facts.html.

34. Hotez PJ, Peiperl L (2015) Noncommunicable diseases: A globalization of disparity? PLOS Med 12(7): e1001859.

35. World Health Organization (2014) Global status report on non-communicable diseases, 2014, http://www.who.int/nmh/publications/ncd-status-report-2014/en.

36. Hosseinpoor AR, Bergen N, Mendis S, Harper S, Verdes E, Kunst A, Chatterji S (2012) Socioeconomic inequality in the prevalence of noncommunicable diseases in low- and middle-income countries: Results from the World Health Survey. BMC Public Health 12:474; doi: 10.1186/1471-2458-12-474.

37. Qui HQ, Rentfro AR, Lu Y, Nair S, Hanis CL, McCormick JB, Fisher-Hoch SP (2012) Host susceptibility to tuberculosis: Insights from a longitudinal study of gene expression in diabetes. Int J Tuberc Lung Dis 16(3): 370–72; doi: 10.5588/ijtld .11.0536.

38. Pang J, Salim A, Lee VJ, Hibberd ML, Chia KS, Leo YS, Lye DC (2012) Diabetes with hypertension as risk factors for adult dengue hemorrhagic fever in a predominantly serotype 2 epidemic: A case control study. PLOS Negl Trop Dis 6(5): e1641.

Chapter 4. East Asia

1. http://www.worldbank.org/en/country/china/overview.

2. http://data.worldbank.org/indicator/SI.POV.DDAY.

3. http://data.worldbank.org/indicator/SI.POV.2DAY/countries.

4. http://www.theglobeandmail.com/news/world/china-building-a-supercity -six-times-bigger-than-nyc/article25590569.

5. Hotez PJ (2012) Engaging a rising China through neglected tropical diseases. PLOS Negl Trop Dis 6(11): e1599; doi:10.1371/journal.pntd.0001599.

6. Coordinating Office of the National Survey on the Important Human Parasitic Diseases (2005) A national survey on current status of the important parasitic diseases in human population (in Chinese). Chin J Parasitol Parasit Dis 23: 332–40.

7. Lai Y-S, Zhou X-N, Utzinger J, Vounatsou P (2013) Bayesian geostatistical modelling of soil-transmitted helminth survey data in the People's Republic of China. Parasites & Vectors 6: 359.

8. Hotez P (2008) Hookworm and poverty. Ann NY Acad Sci 1136: 38–44.

9. Lu L, Liu C, Zhang L, Medina A, Smith S, Rozelle S (2015) Gut instincts: Knowledge, attitudes, and practices regarding soil-transmitted helminths in rural China. PLOS Negl Trop Dis 9(3): e0003643; doi:10.1371/journal.pntd.0003643.

10. Liu C, Luo R, Yi H, Zhang L, Li S, Bai Y, et al. (2015) Soil-transmitted helminths in southwestern China: A cross-sectional study of links to cognitive ability, nutrition, and school performance among children. PLoS Negl Trop Dis 9(6): e0003877.

11. Li S-Z, Zheng H, Abe EM, Yang K, Bergquist R, Qian Y-J, et al. (2014) Reduction patterns of acute schistosomiasis in the People's Republic of China. PLOS Negl Trop Dis 8(5): e2849; doi:10.1371/journal.pntd.0002849.

12. Yang GJ, Liu L, Zhu HR, Griffiths SM, Tanner M, Bergquist R, Utzinger J, Zhou XN (2014) China's sustained drive to eliminate neglected tropical diseases. Lancet Infect Dis 14(9): 881–92.

13. Wang RB, Zhang QF, Zheng B, Xia ZG, Zhou SS, Tang LH, Gao Q, Wang LY, Wang RR (2014) Transition from control to elimination: Impact of the 10-year global fund project on malaria control and elimination in China. Adv Parasitol 86: 289–318.

14. Xia ZG, Zhang L, Feng J, Li M, Feng XY, Tang LH, Wang SQ, Yang HL, Gao Q, Kramer R, Ernest T, Yap P, Zhou XN (2014) Lessons from malaria control to elimination: Case study in Hainan and Yunnan provinces. Adv Parasitol 86: 47–79.

15. Gao X, Nasci R, Liang G (2010) The neglected arboviral infections in mainland China. PLOS Negl Trop Dis 4(4): e624; doi:10.1371/journal.pntd.0000624.

16. Chen J, Zou L, Jin Z, Ruan S (2015) Modeling the geographic spread of rabies in China. PLOS Negl Trop Dis 9(5): e0003772; doi:10.1371/journal.pntd.0003772.

17. World Health Organization (2014) Global status report on non-communicable diseases, http://www.who.int/nmh/publications/ncd-status-report-2014/en.

18. Cai Y (2013) China's new demographic reality: Learning from the 2010 census. Popul Deve Rev 39(3): 371–96.

19. Bethony J, Chen J, Lin S, Xiao S, Zhan B, Li S, Xue H, Xing F, Humphries D, Yan W, Chen G, Foster V, Hawdon JM, Hotez PJ (2002) Emerging patterns of hookworm infection: Influence of aging on the intensity of Necator infection in Hainan Province, People's Republic of China. Clin Infect Dis 35(11) (December 1): 1336–44.

20. http://data.worldbank.org/country/indonesia.

21. Tan M, Kusriastuti R, Savioli L, Hotez PJ (2014) Indonesia: An emerging market economy beset by neglected tropical diseases (NTDs). PLOS Negl Trop Dis 8(2): e2449.

22. http://www.who.int/neglected_diseases/preventive_chemotherapy/sth/en.

23. http://www.who.int/neglected_diseases/preventive_chemotherapy/lf/en.

24. Supali T, Djuardi Y, Bradley M, Noordin R, Rückert P, et al. (2013) Impact of six rounds of mass drug administration on brugian filariasis and soil-transmitted helminth infections in eastern Indonesia. PLOS Negl Trop Dis 7(12): e2586.

25. Bhatt S, Gething PW, Brady OJ, Messina JP, et al. (2013) The global distribution and burden of dengue. Nature 496: 504–7.

26. Shepard DS, Undurraga EA, Halasa YA (2013) Economic and disease burden of dengue in southeast Asia. PLOS Negl Trop Dis 7: e2055.

27. Takeuchi T, Nozaki S, Crump A (2007) Past successes show the way to accomplish future goals. Trends Parasitol 23: 260–67.

28. Humphreys M (2001) Malaria: Poverty, race and public health in the United States. Baltimore, MD: Johns Hopkins University Press.

29. Hotez P (2002) China's hookworms. China Quarterly 172: 1029–41.

30. Ohta N, Waikagul J (2007) Disease burden and epidemiology of soil-transmitted helminthiases and schistosomiasis in Asia: The Japanese perspective. Trends Parasitol 23: 30–35.

31. Ichimori K, Graves PM, Crump A (2007) Lymphatic filariasis elimination in the Pacific: PacELF replicating Japanese successes. Trends Parasitol 23: 54–57.

32. Hong S-T, Chai J-Y, Choi M-H, Huh S, Rim H-J, Lee S-Y (2006) A successful experience of soil-transmitted helminth control in the Republic of Korea. Korean J Parasitol 44: 177–85.

33. Iwagami M, Fukumoto M, Hwang SY, Kim SH, Kho WG, Kano S (2012) Population structure and transmission dynamics of Plasmodium vivax in the Republic of Korea based on microsatellite DNA analysis. PLOS Negl Trop Dis 6(4): e1592.

34. Li S, Shen C, Choi MH, Bae YM, Yoon H, Hong ST (2006) Status of intestinal helminthic infections of borderline residents in North Korea. Korean J Parasitol 44(3): 265–68.

35. Shen C, Li S, Zheng S, Choi MH, Bae YM, Hong ST (2007) Tissue parasitic helminthiases are prevalent at Cheongjin, North Korea. Korean J Parasitol 45(2) (June): 139–44.

36. Kim JE (2014) Nutritional state of children in the Democratic People's Republic of Korea (DPRK): Based on the DPRK final report of the national nutrition survey 2012. Pediatr Gastroenterol Hepatol Nutr. 17(3) (September): 135–39.

37. Linton JA, Tan B, Casey M (2008) A review of tuberculosis prevention, diagnosis and treatment system in the Democratic People's Republic of Korea (DPRK). Asia Pac J Public Health. 20 Suppl (October): 148–55.

38. Hotez PJ (2014) Ten global "hotspots" for the neglected tropical diseases. PLOS Negl Trop Dis 8(5): e2496.

Chapter 5. India

1. http://www.mapsofindia.com/economy.

2. http://data.worldbank.org/indicator/SI.POV.DDAY._

3. http://data.worldbank.org/indicator/SI.POV.2DAY._

4. Lobo DA, Velayudhan R, Chatterjee P, Kohli H, Hotez PJ (2011) The neglected tropical diseases of India and South Asia: Review of their prevalence, distribution, and control or elimination. PLOS Negl Trop Dis 5(10): e1222.

5. http://mapsofindia.com/maps/india/poverty.html.

6. Hotez PJ, Herricks JR (2015) Helminth elimination in the pursuit of sustainable development goals: A "worm index" for human development. PLoS Negl Trop Dis 9(4): e0003618; doi:10.1371/journal.pntd.0003618.

7. Hotez PJ, Brooker S, Bethony JM, Bottazzi ME, Loukas A, Xiao SH (2004) Hookworm infection. N Engl J Med 351: 799–807.

8. http://www.who.int/neglected_diseases/preventive_chemotherapy/sth/en.

9. Greenland K, Dixon R, Khan SA, Gunawardena K, Kihara JH, Smith JL, et al. (2015) The epidemiology of soil-transmitted helminths in Bihar State, India. PLOS Negl Trop Dis 9(5): e0003790.

10. Awasthi S, Peto R, Pande VK, Fletcher RH, Read S, et al. (2008) Effects of deworming on malnourished preschool children in India: An open-labelled, cluster-randomized trial. PLOS Negl Trop Dis 2(4): e223.

11. http://www.who.int/neglected_diseases/preventive_chemotherapy/lf/en.

12. Ramaiah KD, Das PK, Michael E, Guyatt II (2000) The economic burden of lymphatic filariasis in India. Parasitol Today 16(6): 251–53.

13. Babu BV, Mishra S, Nayak AN (2009) Marriage, sex, and hydrocele: An ethnographic study on the effect of filarial hydrocele on conjugal life and marriageability from Orissa, India. PLOS Negl Trop Dis 3(4): e414.

14. Ramaiah KD, Ottesen EA (2014) Progress and impact of 13 years of the Global Programme to Eliminate Lymphatic Filariasis on reducing the burden of filarial disease. PLoS Negl Trop Dis 8(11): e3319.

15. Swaminathan S, Perumal V, Adinarayanan S, Kaliannagounder K, Rengachari R, et al. (2012) Epidemiological assessment of eight rounds of mass drug administration for lymphatic filariasis in India: Implications for monitoring and evaluation. PLOS Negl Trop Dis 6(11): e1926.

16. Addiss DG (2013) Global elimination of lymphatic filariasis: A "mass uprising of compassion." PLOS Negl Trop Dis 7(8): e2264.

17. Budge PJ, Little KM, Mues KE, Kennedy ED, Prakash A, et al. (2013) Impact of community-based lymphedema management on perceived disability among patients with lymphatic filariasis in Orissa State, India. PLOS Negl Trop Dis 7(3): e2100.

18. World Health Organization (2014) Global leprosy update, 2013: Reducing disease burden. Weekly Epidemiol Rec 36(89): 389–400.

19. Jacob JT, Franco-Paredes C (2008) The stigmatization of leprosy in India and its impact on future approaches to elimination and control. PLOS Negl Trop Dis 2(1): e113.

20. Hotez PJ (2013) Forgotten people, forgotten diseases: The neglected tropical diseases and their impact on global health and development, 2nd ed. Washington, DC: ASM Press.

21. Gwalani P (2015) Focus on India in fight against neglected tropical diseases. Times of India, April 9, http://timesofindia.indiatimes.com/city/nagpur/Focus-on -India-in-fight-against-neglected-tropical-diseases/articleshow/46856862.cms.

22. John TJ, Dandona L, Sharma VP, Kakkar M (2011) Continuing challenge of infectious diseases in India. Lancet 377: 252–69.

23. Hotez P (2014) World Health Day. Huffington Post, April 2, http://www.huff ingtonpost.com/peter-hotez-md-phd/post_7254_b_5072181.html.

24. Singh PK, Dhiman RC (2012) Climate change and human health: Indian context. J Vector Borne Dis 49: 55–60.

25. Alvar J, Velez IV, Bern C, Herrero M, Desjeux P, Cano J, Jannin J, den Boer M, the WHO Leishmaniasis Control Team. 2012. Leishmaniasis worldwide and global estimates of its incidence. PLOS One 7: e35671.

26. Burza S, Sinha PK, Mahajan R, Lima MA, Mitra G, et al. (2014) Five-year field results and long-term effectiveness of 20 mg/kg liposomal amphotericin B (Ambisome) for visceral leishmaniasis in Bihar, India. PLOS Negl Trop Dis 8(1): e2603.

27. http://nvbdcp.gov.in/kal2.html.

28. http://www.gilead.com/responsibility/developing-world-access/visceral%20 leishmaniasis.

29. http://www.doctorswithoutborders.org/news-stories/press-release/msf -statement-response-gilead-donation-ambisome-visceral-leishmaniasis.

30. Sundar S, Singh A, Rai M, Chakravarty J (2015) Single-dose indigenous liposomal amphotericin B in the treatment of Indian visceral leishmaniasis: A phase 2 study. Am J Trop Med Hyg 92(3): 513–17.

31. Coleman M, Foster GM, Deb R, Pratap Singh R, Ismail HM, Shivam P, Ghosh AK, Dunkley S, Kumar V, Coleman M, Hemingway J, Paine MJ, Das P (2015) DDT-based indoor residual spraying suboptimal for visceral leishmaniasis elimination in India. Proc Natl Acad Sci U S A 112(28): 8573–78.

32. Dhingra N, Jha P, Sharma VP, Cohen AA, Jotkar RM, Rodriguez PS, Bassani DG, Suraweera W, Laxminarayan R, Peto R, Million Death Study Collaborators (2010) Adult and child malaria mortality in India: A nationally representative mortality survey. Lancet 376: 1768–74.

33. Hotez PJ (2015) Blue marble health and "the big three diseases": HIV/AIDS, tuberculosis, and malaria. Microbes Infec [Epub ahead of print].

34. Bhatt S, Gething PW, Brady OJ, Messina JP, et al. (2013) The global distribution and burden of dengue. Nature 496: 504–7.

35. Harris G (2012) As dengue fever sweeps India, a slow response stirs experts' fears. New York Times, November 6.

36. Kumar A, Chery L, Biswas C, Nubhashi N, Dutta P, et al. (2012) Malaria in South Asia: Prevalence and control. Acta Trop 121(3): 246–55.

37. Kakkar M, Venkataramanan V, Krishnan S, Chauhan RS, Abbas SS (2012) Moving from rabies research to rabies control: Lessons from India. PLOS Negl Trop Dis 6(8): e1748.

38. Mohapatra B, Warrell DA, Suraweera W, Bhatia P, Dhingra N, et al. (2011) Snakebite mortality in India: A nationally representative mortality survey. PLOS Negl Trop Dis 5(4): e1018.

39. Abd El Ghany M, Chander J, Mutreja A, Rashid M, Hill-Cawthorne GA, et al. (2014) The population structure of Vibrio cholerae from the Chandigarh region of northern India. PLOS Negl Trop Dis 8(7): e2981.

40. Hotez PJ, Peiperl L (2015) Non-communicable diseases: A globalization of disparity? PLOS Medicine 12(7): e1001859.

41. Burki T (2015) Why India should worry about a coepidemic of diabetes and tuberculosis. BMJ 350: h111.

42. Basu S, Millett C, Vijan S, Hayward RA, Kinra S, Ahuja R, et al. (2015) The health system and population health implications of large-scale diabetes screening in India: A microsimulation model of alternative approaches. PLOS Med 12(5): e1001827.

43. Raghuraman S, Vasudevan KP, Govindarajan S, Chinnakali P, Panigrahi KC (2014) Prevalence of diabetes mellitus among tuberculosis patients in urban Puducherry. N Am J Med Sci 6(1): 30–34.

44. Karunakaran A, Ilyas WM, Sheen SF, Jose NK, Nujum ZT (2014) Risk factors of mortality among dengue patients admitted to a tertiary care setting in Kerala, India. J Infect Public Health 7(2) (March–April): 114–20; doi: 10.1016/j.jiph.2013.09.006.

45. Babu S, Salve H, Krishnan A (2013) Tuberculosis and diabetes mellitus: Time for an integrated approach. Natl Med J India 26(6): 342–43.

46. Lakshman N (2011) India facing heavy burden of neglected tropical diseases. Hindu, November 1, http://www.thehindu.com/news/national/article2587921.ece.

47. Hotez PJ (2010) Nuclear weapons and neglected diseases: The "ten-thousand -to-one gap." PLOS Negl Trop Dis 4(4): e680.

Chapter 6. Sub-Saharan Africa

1. Molyneux DH, Hotez PJ, Fenwick A (2005) "Rapid-impact interventions": How a policy of integrated control for Africa's neglected tropical diseases could benefit the poor. PLOS Med 2(11): e336.

2. World Health Organization (2015) Planning, requesting medicines and reporting for preventive chemotherapy. Weekly Epidemiol Rec 90(14): 133–48.

3. http://www.worldbank.org/en/region/afr/overview.

4. https://www.elliottwave.com/freeupdates/archives/2011/02/09/Surprising-Economic-Path-for-the--Forgotten-Continent-.aspx.

5. http://data.worldbank.org/topic/poverty.

6. http://data.worldbank.org/indicator/SI.POV.DDAY.

7. Hotez P (2013) South Sudan's forgotten people and their forgotten diseases. Huffington Post, December 31, http://www.huffingtonpost.com/peter-hotez-md-phd/south-sudans-forgotten-pe_b_4524653.html.

8. Hotez PJ (2015) Neglected tropical diseases in the Ebola-affected countries of West Africa. PLOS Negl Trop Dis 9(6): e0003671.

9. Hotez PJ, Molyneux DH (2008) Tropical anemia: One of Africa's great killers and a rationale for linking malaria and neglected tropical disease control to achieve a common goal. PLOS Negl Trop Dis 2(7): e270.

10. Hotez PJ, Ferris MT (2006) The antipoverty vaccines. Vaccine 24(31–32): 5787–99.

11. http://www.afdb.org/en/countries/west-africa/nigeria/nigeria-economic-outlook.

12. http://www.cconomist.com/blogs/economist-explains/2014/04/economist-explains-2.

13. http://data.worldbank.org/indicator/SI.POV.DDAY.

14. http://data.worldbank.org/indicator/SI.POV.2DAY.

15. Hotez PJ, Asojo OA, Adesina AM (2012) Nigeria: "Ground zero" for the high prevalence neglected tropical diseases. PLOS Negl Trop Dis 6(7): e1600.

16. Hotez PJ, Herricks JR (2015) Helminth elimination in the pursuit of sustainable development goals: A "worm index" for human development. PLOS Negl Trop Dis 9(4): e0003618.

17. http://www.who.int/neglected_diseases/preventive_chemotherapy/sth/en.

18. http://www.who.int/neglected_diseases/preventive_chemotherapy/lf/en.

19. http://www.who.int/neglected_diseases/preventive_chemotherapy/sch/en.

20. Hotez PJ (2015) Boko Haram and Africa's neglected tropical diseases. PLOS Speaking of Medicine blog, March 12, http://blogs.plos.org/speakingofmedicine/2015/03/12/boko-haram-africas-neglected-tropical-diseases.

21. http://www.cartercenter.org/countries/nigeria-health-schistosomiasis.html.

22. http://www.cartercenter.org/countries/nigeria-health.html.

23. http://www.neglecteddiseases.gov/countries/nigeria.html.

24. http://www.ntdenvision.org/about_envision.

25. http://www.sightsavers.org/way-elimination-nigeria.

26. http://www.schoolsandhealth.org/News/Pages/Nigeria%20Launches%20Master%20Plan%20for%20Neglected%20Tropical%20Diseases.aspx.

27. http://www.neglecteddiseases.gov/newsroom/voices_from_the_field/johnathan_nigeria.html.

28. Hotez P, Mistry N (2015) The planet's children and their neglected tropical diseases (June), http://www.healio.com/pediatrics/emerging-diseases/news/print

/infectious-diseases-in-children/%7B15f9eb4a-0069-490b-9988-3060ca7d5977%7D
/the-planets-children-and-their-neglected-tropical-diseases.

29. http://www.topuniversities.com/university-rankings/world-university
-rankings/2015#sorting=rank+region=6+country=+faculty=+stars=false+search=.

30. From annex table 3: People living with HIV (all ages), 2005 and 2013, pp. A18–A23. In: UNAIDS. The Gap Report, http://www.unaids.org/en/resources/documents
/2014/20140716_UNAIDS_gap_report.

31. http://www.avert.org/hiv-aids-south-africa.htm.

32. Berge ST, Kabatereine N, Gundersen SG, Taylor M, Kvalsvig JD, Mikhize-Kwitshana Z, Jinabhai C, Kjetland EF (2011) Generic praziquantel in South Africa: The necessity for policy change to provide cheap, safe and efficacious schistosomiasis drugs for the poor, rural population. South African J Infect Dis 26(1): http://www.sajei.co.za/index.php/SAJEI/article/view/302.

33. Kjetland EF, Hegertun IE, Baay MF, Onsrud M, Ndhlovu PD, Taylor M (2014) Genital schistosomiasis and its unacknowledged role on HIV transmission in the STD intervention studies. Int J STD AIDS 25(10): 705–15.

34. Downs JA, van Dam GJ, Changalucha JM, Corstjens PL, Peck RN, de Dood CJ, Bang H, Andreasen A, Kalluvya SE, van Lieshout L, Johnson WD Jr, Fitzgerald DW (2012) Association of schistosomiasis and HIV infection in Tanzania. Am J Trop Med Hyg 87(5): 868–73.

35. Hegertun IE, Sulheim Gundersen KM, Kleppa E, Zulu SG, Gundersen SG, Taylor M, Kvalsvig JD, Kjetland EF (2013) S. haematobium as a common cause of genital morbidity in girls: A cross-sectional study of children in South Africa. PLOS Negl Trop Dis 7(3):e2104.

36. Ndeffo Mbah ML, Poolman EM, Atkins KE, Orenstein EW, Meyers LA, Townsend JP, et al. (2013) Potential cost-effectiveness of schistosomiasis treatment for reducing HIV transmission in Africa: The case of Zimbabwean women. PLOS Negl Trop Dis 7(8): e2346.

37. Hotez PJ, Bethony JM, Diemert DJ, Pearson M, Loukas A (2010) Developing vaccines to combat hookworm infection and intestinal schistosomiasis. Nat Rev Microbiol 8(11): 814–26.

38. Hotez P, Whitham M (2014) Helminth infections: A new global women's health agenda. Obstet Gynecol 123(1): 155–60.

39. McNeil DG Jr (2014) A simple theory, and a proposal, on HIV in Africa. New York Times, May 10, http://www.nytimes.com/2014/05/11/health/a-simple-theory-and-a-proposal-on-hiv-in-africa.html?_r=0.

Chapter 7. Saudi Arabia and Neighboring Conflict Zones of the Middle East and North African Region

1. http://www.theguardian.com/world/2013/jan/01/saudi-arabia-riyadh-poverty
-inequality.

2. Mohammad KA (2014) Prevalence of schistosomiasis in Al-Baha Province, Saudi Arabia in years 2012 and 2013 (prospective and comparative study). J Egypt Soc Parasitol 44(2): 397–404.

3. Salam N, Al-Shaqha WM, Azzi A (2014) Leishmaniasis in the Middle East: Incidence and epidemiology. PLOS Negl Trop Dis 8(10): e3208; doi:10.1371/journal.pntd.0003208.

4. Hotez PJ, Savioli L, Fenwick A (2012) Neglected tropical diseases of the Middle East and North Africa: Review of their prevalence, distribution, and opportunities for control. PLOS Negl Trop Dis 6(2): e1475.

5. Hotez PJ (2009) The neglected tropical diseases and their devastating health and economic impact on the member nations of the Organisation of the Islamic Conference. PLOS Negl Trop Dis 3(10): e539.

6. Azhar EI, Hashem AM, El-Kafrawy SA, Abol-Ela S, Abd-Alla AM, Sohrab SS, Farraj SA, Othman NA, Ben-Helaby HG, Ashshi A, Madani TA, Jamjoom G (2015) Complete genome sequencing and phylogenetic analysis of dengue type 1 virus isolated from Jeddah, Saudi Arabia. Virol J 12 (January 16): 1; doi: 10.1186/s12985 014 0235-7.

7. Aziz AT, Al-Shami SA, Mahyoub JA, Hatabbi M, Ahmad AH, Rawi CS (2014) An update on the incidence of dengue gaining strength in Saudi Arabia and current control approaches for its vector mosquito. Parasit Vectors 7: 258; doi: 10.1186/1756–3305-7-258.

8. Mokdad AH, Jaber S, Aziz MI, AlBuhairan F, AlGhaithi A, AlHamad NM, Al-Hooti SN, et al. (2014) The state of health in the Arab world, 1990–2010: An analysis of the burden of diseases, injuries, and risk factors. Lancet 383(9914): 309–20.

9. Gosadi IM, Goyder EC, Teare MD (2014) Investigating the potential effect of consanguinity on type 2 diabetes susceptibility in a Saudi population. Hum Hered 77(1–4): 197–206.

10. Khan AR, Al Abdul Lateef ZN, Fatima S, Al Yousuf SA, Khan Afghan SZ, Al Marghani S (2014) Prevalence of chronic complication among type 2 diabetics attending primary health care centers of Al Ahsa district of Saudi Arabia: A cross sectional survey. Glob J Health Sci 6(4): 245–53.

11. Karunakaran A, Ilyas WM, Sheen SF, Jose NK, Nujum ZT (2014) Risk factors of mortality among dengue patients admitted to a tertiary care setting in Kerala, India. J Infect Public Health 7(2): 114–20.

12. Hotez PJ (2015) Vaccine science diplomacy: Expanding capacity to prevent emerging and neglected tropical diseases arising from Islamic State (IS)–held territories. PLOS Negl Trop Dis 9(9): e0003852.

13. http://www.worldbank.org/en/region/mena/overview.

14. Bhatt S, Gething PW, Brady OJ, Messina JP, et al. (2013) The global distribution and burden of dengue. Nature 496: 504–7.

15. Bausch DG, Schwarz L (2014) Outbreak of Ebola virus disease in Guinea: Where ecology meets economy. PLOS Negl Trop Dis 8(7): e3056.

16. Hotez PJ (2015) Combating the next lethal epidemic. Science 348(6232): 296–97.

17. GBD 2013 Mortality and Causes of Death Collaborators (2015) Global, regional, and national age-sex specific all-cause and cause-specific mortality for 240 causes of death, 1990–2013: A systematic analysis for the Global Burden of Disease Study 2013. Lancet 385(9963): 117–71.

18. Hotez PJ (2013) "Aleppo evil": The ulcer, the boil, the sandfly, and the conflict. PLOS Speaking of Medicine blog (June 5), http://blogs.plos.org/speakingof medicine/2013/06/05/aleppo-evil-%D9%82%D8%B1%D8%AD%D8%A9-%D8%AD %D9%84%D8%A8-the-ulcer-the-boil-the-sandfly-and-the-conflict.

19. Ben Embarek PK, Van Kerkhova MD, and World Health Organization (2015) Middle East respiratory syndrome coronavirus (MERS-CoV): Current situation 3 years after the virus was first identified. Weekly Epidemiol Rec 90(20): 245–50.

20. http://ecdc.europa.eu/en/press/news/_layouts/forms/News_DispForm.aspx ?ID=1228&List=8db7286c-fe2d-476c-9133-18ff4cb1b568&Source=http2F2Eeuropa 2Fen2Fhome.aspx.

Chapter 8. The Americas

1. http://data.worldbank.org/indicator/SI.POV.GINI.

2. http://www.civicdashboards.com/city/houston-tx-16000US4835000/gini _index.

3. http://www.economist.com/news/ special-report/21564411-unequal-continent-becoming-less-so-gini-back-bottle.

4. http://www.worldbank.org/en/region/lac/overview.

5. Hotez PJ, Dumonteil E, Heffernan MJ, Bottazzi ME (2013) Innovation for the "bottom 100 million": Eliminating neglected tropical diseases in the Americas. Adv Exp Med Biol 764: 1–12.

6. Pullan RL, Smith JL, Jasrasaria R, Brooker SJ (2014) Global numbers of infection and disease burden of soil transmitted helminth infections in 2010. Parasit Vectors 7: 37.

7. World Health Organization (2015) Chagas disease in Latin America: An epidemiological update based on 2010 estimates. Weekly Epidemiol Rec 90(6): 33–44.

8. http://www.who.int/neglected_diseases/preventive_chemotherapy/sch/en.

9. http://www.who.int/malaria/publications/world_malaria_report_2014/wmr -2014-regional-profiles.pdf?ua=1.

10. http://data.worldbank.org/country.

11. http://www.who.int/neglected_diseases/preventive_chemotherapy/sth/en.

12. http://data.worldbank.org/country/argentina.

13. http://krugman.blogs.nytimes.com/?s=argentina&_r=0.

14. Hotez PJ (2014) Ten global "hotspots" for the neglected tropical diseases. PLOS Negl Trop Dis 8(5): e2496; doi:10.1371/journal.pntd.0002496.

15. Vazquez-Prokopec GM, Spillmann C, Zaidenberg M, Kitron U, Gürtler RE (2009) Cost-effectiveness of Chagas disease vector control strategies in northwestern Argentina. PLOS Negl Trop Dis 3(1): e363.

16. Gürtler RE, Cecere MC, Fernández MdP, Vazquez-Prokopec GM, Ceballos LA, Gurevitz JM, et al. (2014) Key source habitats and potential dispersal of Triatoma infestans populations in northwestern Argentina: Implications for vector control. PLOS Negl Trop Dis 8(10): e3238.

17. http://www.mundosano.org/en.

18. http://www.worldbank.org/en/country/brazil/overview.

19. http://www.nytimes.com/2015/08/09/business/international/effects-of-petro bras-scandal-leave-brazilians-lamenting-a-lost-dream.html?_r=0.

20. http://data.worldbank.org/indicator/SI.POV.2DAY.

21. Hotez PJ, Fujiwara RT (2014) Brazil's neglected tropical diseases: An overview and a report card. Microbes Infect 16(8): 601–6.

22. Sarvel AK, Oliveira ÁA, Silva AR, Lima ACL, Katz N (2011) Evaluation of a 25-year-program for the control of schistosomiasis mansoni in an endemic area in Brazil. PLOS Negl Trop Dis 5(3): e990.

23. Rodriguez-Barraquer I, Cordeiro MT, Braga C, de Souza WV, Marques ET, Cummings DAT (2011) From re-emergence to hyperendemicity: The natural history of the dengue epidemic in Brazil. PLOS Negl Trop Dis 5(1): e935.

24. Villabona-Arenas CJ, de Oliveira JL, Capra CdS, Balarini K, Loureiro M, Fonseca CRTP, et al. (2014) Detection of four dengue serotypes suggests rise in hyperendemicity in urban centers of Brazil. PLOS Negl Trop Dis 8(2): e2620.

25. van Panhuis WG, Hyun S, Blaney K, Marques ETA Jr, Coelho GE, Siqueira JB Jr, et al. (2014) Risk of dengue for tourists and teams during the World Cup 2014 in Brazil. PLOS Negl Trop Dis 8(7): e3063.

26. http://www.paho.org/hq/index.php?option=com_topics&view=article&id= 427&Itemid=41484&lang=en.

27. http://www.cdts.fiocruz.br/cdts/ingles.

28. http://www.worldbank.org/en/country/mexico/overview.

29. Hotez PJ, Bottazzi ME, Dumonteil E, Valenzuela JG, Kamhawi S, Ortega J, et al. (2012) Texas and Mexico: Sharing a legacy of poverty and neglected tropical diseases. PLOS Negl Trop Dis 6(3): e1497.

30. Hotez PJ, Bottazzi ME, Dumonteil E, Buekens P (2015) The Gulf of Mexico: A "hot zone" for neglected tropical diseases? PLOS Negl Trop Dis 9(2): e0003481.

31. Fleury A, Moreno García J, Valdez Aguerrebere P, de Sayve Durán M, Becerril Rodríguez P, Larralde C, et al. (2010) Neurocysticercosis, a persisting health problem in Mexico. PLOS Negl Trop Dis 4(8): e805.

32. Bhattarai R, Budke CM, Carabin H, Proaño JV, Flores Rivera J, Corona T, et al. (2012) Estimating the non-monetary burden of neurocysticercosis in Mexico. PLOS Negl Trop Dis 6(2): e1521.

33. Flisser A, Correa D (2010) Neurocysticercosis may no longer be a public health problem in Mexico. PLOS Negl Trop Dis 4(12): e831.

34. Hotez PJ, Dumonteil E, Betancourt Cravioto M, Bottazzi ME, Tapia-Conyer R, Meymandi S, et al. (2013) An unfolding tragedy of Chagas disease in North America. PLOS Negl Trop Dis 7(10): e2300.

35. Cruz-Reyes A, Pickering-Lopez JM (2006) Chagas disease in Mexico: An analysis of geographical distribution during the past 76 years—a review. Mem Inst Oswaldo Cruz, Rio de Janiero 101(4): 345–54.

36. Manne JM, Snively CS, Ramsey JM, Salgado MO, Bärnighausen T, Reich MR (2013) Barriers to treatment access for Chagas disease in Mexico. PLOS Negl Trop Dis 7(10): e2488.

37. Ramsey JM, Elizondo-Cano M, Sanchez-González G, Peña-Nieves A, Figueroa-Lara A (2014) Opportunity cost for early treatment of Chagas disease in Mexico. PLOS Negl Trop Dis 8(4): e2776.

38. Hotez PJ, Dumonteil E, Woc-Colburn L, Serpa JA, Bezek S, Edwards MS, et al. (2012) Chagas disease: "The new HIV/AIDS of the Americas." PLOS Negl Trop Dis 6(5): e1498.

39. Undurraga EA, Betancourt-Cravioto M, Ramos-Castañeda J, Martínez-Vega R, Méndez-Galván J, Gubler DJ, et al. (2015) Economic and disease burden of dengue in Mexico. PLOS Negl Trop Dis 9(3): e0003547.

40. http://www.carlosslim.com/responsabilidad_ing.html.

Chapter 9. Australia, Canada, European Union, Russian Federation, and Turkey

1. Hotez PJ (2014) Aboriginal populations and their neglected tropical diseases. PLOS Negl Trop Dis 8(1): e2286.

2. Kline K, McCarthy JS, Pearson M, Loukas A, Hotez PJ (2013) Neglected tropical diseases of Oceania: Review of their prevalence, distribution, and opportunities for control. PLOS Negl Trop Dis 7(1): e1755.

3. Davis JS, McGloughlin S, Tong SYC, Walton SF, Currie BJ (2013) A novel clinical grading scale to guide the management of crusted scabies. PLOS Negl Trop Dis 7(9): e2387.

4. Engelman D, Kiang K, Chosidow O, McCarthy J, Fuller C, Lammie P, Hay R, Steer A; Members of the International Alliance for the Control of Scabies (2013) Toward the global control of human scabies: Introducing the International Alliance for the Control of Scabies. PLOS Negl Trop Dis 7(8): e2167.

5. Ginther JL, Mayo M, Warrington SD, Kaestli M, Mullins T, Wagner DM, et al. (2015) Identification of Burkholderia pseudomallei near-neighbor species in the Northern Territory of Australia. PLOS Negl Trop Dis 9(6): e0003892.

6. Shattock AJ, Gambhir M, Taylor HR, Cowling CS, Kaldor JM, Wilson DP (2015) Control of trachoma in Australia: A model-based evaluation of current interventions. PLOS Negl Trop Dis 9(4): e0003474.

7. Lavender CJ, Fyfe JAM, Azuolas J, Brown K, Evans RN, Ray LR, et al. (2011) Risk of Buruli ulcer and detection of Mycobacterium ulcerans in mosquitoes in southeastern Australia. PLOS Negl Trop Dis 5(9): e1305.

8. Hotez PJ, Velasquez RM, Wolf JE Jr (2014) Neglected tropical skin diseases: Their global elimination through integrated mass drug administration. JAMA Dermatol 150(5): 481–82.

9. Hotez PJ (2010) Neglected infections of poverty among the indigenous peoples of the Arctic. PLOS Negl Trop Dis 4(1): e606.

10. Schurer JM, Rafferty E, Farag M, Zeng W, Jenkins EJ (2015) Echinococcosis: An economic evaluation of a veterinary public health intervention in rural Canada. PLOS Negl Trop Dis 9(7): e0003883.

11. Elmore SA, Jenkins EJ, Huyvaert KP, Polley L, Root JJ, Moore CG (2012) Toxoplasma gondii in circumpolar people and wildlife. Vector Borne Zoonotic Dis 12(1): 1–9.

12. Schurer JM, Ndao M, Skinner S, Irvine J, Elmore SA, Epp T, et al. (2013) Parasitic zoonoses: One health surveillance in northern Saskatchewan. PLOS Negl Trop Dis 7(3): e2141.

13. Hueffer K, Parkinson AJ, Gerlach R, Berner J (2013) Zoonotic infections in Alaska: Disease prevalence, potential impact of climate change and recommended actions for earlier disease detection, research, prevention and control. Int J Circumpolar Health 72: doi: 10.3402/ijch.v72i0.19562.

14. Parkinson AJ, Evengard B, Semenza JC, Ogden N, Børresen ML, Berner J, Brubaker M, et al. (2014) Climate change and infectious diseases in the Arctic: Establishment of a circumpolar working group. Int J Circumpolar Health 73: 25163.

15. Himsworth CG, Bidulka J, Parsons KL, Feng AYT, Tang P, Jardine CM, et al. (2013) Ecology of Leptospira interrogans in Norway rats (Rattus norvegicus) in an inner-city neighborhood of Vancouver, Canada. PLOS Negl Trop Dis 7(6): e2270.

16. http://data.worldbank.org/region/EUU.

17. Le Bailly M, Landolt M, Bouchet F (2012) First World War German soldier intestinal worms: An original study of trench latrine in France. J Parasitol 98(6): 1273–75.

18. Bøås H, Tapia G, Sødahl JA, Rasmussen T, Rønningen KS (2012) Enterobius vermicularis and risk factors in healthy Norwegian children. Pediatr Infect Dis J 31(9): 927–30.

19. Del Brutto OH (2012) Neurocysticercosis in western Europe: A re-emerging disease? Acta Neurol Belg 112(4): 335–43.

20. Fabiani S, Bruschi F (2013) Neurocysticercosis in Europe: Still a public health concern not only for imported cases. Acta Trop 128(1): 18–26.

21. Schneider R, Aspock H, Auer H (2013) Unexpected increase of alveolar echinococcosis, Austria, 2011. Emerg Infect Dis 19(3): 475–77.

22. Hotez PJ, Gurwith M (2011) Europe's neglected infections of poverty. Int J Infect Dis 15(9): e611–19.

23. Neghina R, Dumitrascu V, Neghina AM, Vlad DC, Petrica L, Vermesan D, Tirnea L, Mazilu O, Olariu TR (2013) Epidemiology of ascariasis, enterobiasis and giardiasis in a Romanian western county (Timis), 1993–2006. Acta Trop 125(1) (January): 98–101

24. Sejdini A, Mahmud R, Lim YA, Mahdy M, Sejdini F, Gjoni V, Xhaferraj K, Kasmi G. (2011) Intestinal parasitic infections among children in central Albania. Ann Trop Med Parasitol 105(3) (April): 241–50.

25. Gołąb E, Czarkowski MP (2014) Echinococcosis and cysticercosis in Poland in 2012. Przegl Epidemiol 68(2): 279–82, 379–81.

26. Šoba B, Beović B, Lužnik Z, Skvarč M, Logar J (2014) Evidence of human neurocysticercosis in Slovenia. Parasitology 141(4) (April): 547–53.

27. Czarkowski MP, Gołab E (2013) Invasive tapeworm infections in Poland in 2011. Przegl Epidemiol 67(2): 263–66, 365–67.

28. Antolova D, Miterpakova M, Radoňak J, Hudačkova D, Szilagyiova M, Začek M (2014) Alveolar echinococcosis in a highly endemic area of northern Slovakia between 2000 and 2013. Euro Surveill 19(34): pii: 20882.

29. Dobrescu C, Hriscu H, Emandi M, Zamfir C, Nemet C (2014) Consumption of untested pork contributed to over two thousand clinical cases of human trichinellosis in Romania. Folia Parasitol (Praha) 61(6): 558–60.

30. Sadkowska-Todys M, Gołab E (2013) Trichinellosis in Poland in 2011. Przegl Epidemiol 67(2): 259–61, 363–64.

31. Schaffner F, Mathis A (2014) Dengue and dengue vectors in the WHO European region: Past, present, and scenarios for the future. Lancet Infect Dis 14(12): 1271–80.

32. Di Sabatino D, Bruno R, Sauro F, Danzetta ML, Cito F, Iannetti S, Narcisi V, De Massis F, Calistri P (2014) Epidemiology of West Nile disease in Europe and in the Mediterranean basin from 2009 to 2013. Biomed Res Int 2014: 907852.

33. Pupella S, Pisani G, Cristiano K, Catalano L, Grazzini G (2014) Update on West Nile virus in Italy. Blood Transfus 12(4): 626–27.

34. Tomasello D, Schlagenhauf P (2013) Chikungunya and dengue autochthonous cases in Europe, 2007–2012. Travel Med Infect Dis 11(5): 274–84.

35. Papa A, Sidira P, Larichev V, Gavrilova L, Kuzmina K, Mousavi-Jazi M, Mirazimi A, Stroher U, Nichol S (2014) Crimean-Congo hemorrhagic fever virus, Greece. Emerg Infect Dis 20(2): 288–90.

36. Valerio L, Roure S, Fernández-Rivas G, Basile L, Martínez-Cuevas O, Ballesteros ÁL, Ramos X, Sabrià M; North Metropolitan Working Group on Imported Diseases (2013) Strongyloides stercoralis, the hidden worm. Epidemiological and clinical characteristics of 70 cases diagnosed in the North Metropolitan Area of Barcelona, Spain, 2003–2012. Trans R Soc Trop Med Hyg 107(8): 465–70.

37. Glize B, Malvy D (2014) Autochthonous strongyloidiasis, Bordeaux area, south-western France.Travel Med Infect Dis 12(1): 106–8.

38. Pozio E, Armignacco O, Ferri F, Gomez Morales MA (2013) Opisthorchis felineus, an emerging infection in Italy and its implication for the European Union. Acta Trop 126(1): 54–62.

39. de Laval F, Savini H, Biance-Valero E, Simon F (2014) Human schistosomiasis: An emerging threat for Europe. Lancet 384(9948): 1094–95.

40. Salvador F, Treviño B, Sulleiro E, Pou D, Sánchez-Montalvá A, Cabezos J, Soriano A, et al. (2014) Trypanosoma cruzi infection in a non-endemic country: Epidemiological and clinical profile. Clin Microbiol Infect 20(7): 706–12.

41. Antoniou M, Gramiccia M, Molina AR, Dvorak V, Volf P (2013) The role of indigenous phlebotomine sandflies in mammals in the spreading of leishmaniasis agents in the Mediterranean region. Euro Surveill 18(30): 20540.

42. Fros JJ, Geertsema C, Vogels CB, Roosjen PP, Failloux A-B, Vlak JM, et al. (2015) West Nile virus: High transmission rate in north-western European mosquitoes indicates its epidemic potential and warrants increased surveillance. PLOS Negl Trop Dis 9(7): e0003956.

43. Hotez PJ, Papageorgiou TD (2013) A new European Neglected Diseases Center for Greece? PLOS Negl Trop Dis 7(2): e1757.

44. Semenza JC, Sudre B, Oni T, Suk JE, Giesecke J (2013) Linking environmental drivers to infectious diseases: The European Environment and Epidemiology Network. PLOS Negl Trop Dis 7(7): e2323.

45. Gallup JL, Sachs JD (2001) The economic burden of malaria. Am J Trop Med Hyg 64(1–2 Suppl): 85–96.

46. Hotez PJ (2015) A new wave of diseases threatens southern Europe and the Middle East. Washington Post, October 23, https://www.washingtonpost.com /opinions/preventing-the-next-disease-outbreaks/2015/10/23/c4564ec0-7817-11e5 -a958-d889faf561dc_story.html.

47. http://www.worldbank.org/en/country/russia/overview.

48. http://www.themoscowtimes.com/business/article/putin-era-prosperity-fades -as-more-russians-slip-into-poverty/523422.html.

49. Baranova AM, Ezhov MN, Guzeeva TM, Morozova LF (2013) The current malaria situation in the CIS countries (2011–2012) (in Russian). Med Parazitol (Mosk) (4): 7–10.

50. Onishchenko GG, Lipnitskiĭ AV, Alekseev VV, Antonov VA, Kriuchkova TP, Krutogolovova TA (2011) Epidemiologic situation of West Nile fever in Russia in 2010 (in Russian). Zh Mikrobiol Epidemiol Immunobiol (3): 115–20.

51. Konyaev SV, Yanagida T, Nakao M, Ingovatova GM, Shoykhet YN, Bondarev AY, Odnokurtsev VA, et al. (2013) Genetic diversity of Echinococcus spp. in Russia. Parasitology 140(13): 1637–47.

52. Kuchta R, Brabec J, Kubáčková P, Scholz T (2013) Tapeworm Diphyllobothrium dendriticum (Cestoda)—neglected or emerging human parasite? PLOS Negl Trop Dis 7(12): e2535.

53. Ogorodova LM, Fedorova OS, Sripa B, Mordvinov VA, Katokhin AV, Keiser J, et al. (2015) Opisthorchiasis: An overlooked danger. PLOS Negl Trop Dis 9(4): e0003563.

54. Mordvinov VA, Yurlova NI, Ogorodova LM, Katokhin AV (2012) Opisthorchis felineus and Metorchis bilis are the main agents of liver fluke infection of humans in Russia. Parasitol Int 61(1): 25–31.

55. http://www.worldbank.org/en/country/turkey/overview.

56. http://data.worldbank.org/indicator/SI.POV.2DAY.

57. Özbilgina A, Topluoglu S, Es S, Islek E, Mollahaliloglu S, Erkoc Y (2011) Malaria in Turkey: Successful control and strategies for achieving elimination. Acta Trop 120(1–2): 15–23.

58. Gürel MS, Yeşilova Y, Olgen MK, Ozbel Y (2012) Cutaneous leishmaniasis in Turkey (in Turkish). Turkiye Parazitol Derg 36(2): 121–29.

59. Kırkoyun Uysal H, Akgül O, Purisa S, Oner YA (2014) Twenty-five years of intestinal parasite prevalence in İstanbul University, İstanbul Faculty of Medicine: A retrospective study (in Turkish). Turkiye Parazitol Derg 38(2): 97–101.

60. Çevik M, Eser I, Boleken ME (2013) Characteristics and outcomes of liver and lung hydatid disease in children. Trop Doct 43(3): 93–95.

61. Yumuk Z, O'Callaghan D (2012) Brucellosis in Turkey—an overview. Int J Infect Dis 16(4): e228–35.

62. Ergunay K, Gunay F, Erisoz Kasap O, Oter K, Gargari S, Karaoglu T, et al. (2014) Serological, molecular and entomological surveillance demonstrates widespread circulation of West Nile virus in Turkey. PLOS Negl Trop Dis 8(7): e3028.

63. Orkun Ö, Karaer Z, Çakmak A, Nalbantoğlu S (2014) Identification of tick-borne pathogens in ticks feeding on humans in Turkey. PLOS Negl Trop Dis 8(8): e3067.

64. http://data.unhcr.org/syrianrefugees/regional.php.

Chapter 10. United States of America

1. Hotez PJ, Ferris MT (2006) The antipoverty vaccines. Vaccine 24(31–32): 5787–99.

2. Hotez PJ, Fenwick A, Savioli L, Molyneux DH (2009) Rescuing the bottom billion through control of neglected tropical diseases. Lancet 373(9674): 1570–75.

3. Harrington M (1962) The other America: Poverty in the United States. New York: Penguin Books, pp 1–2.

4. http://www.census.gov/newsroom/press-releases/2014/cb14–169.html.

5. Shaefer HL, Edin K (2013) Rising extreme poverty in the United States and the response of federal means-tested transfer programs, http://npc.umich.edu/publications/working_papers/?publication_id=255&.

6. Denavas-Walt C, Proctor BD, Smith JC, US Census Bureau (2011) Income, poverty, and health insurance coverage in the United States: 2010, http://www.census.gov/prod/2011pubs/p60–239.pdf.

7. Abramsky S (2013) The American way of poverty: How the other half still lives. New York: Nation Books.

8. Hotez PJ (2008) Neglected infections of poverty in the United States of America. PLOS Negl Trop Dis 2(6): e256.

9. Hotez PJ (2014) Neglected parasitic infections and poverty in the United States. PLOS Negl Trop Dis 8(9): e3012.

10. Glasmeier AK (2006) An atlas of poverty in America: One nation, pulling apart, 1960–2003. New York: Routledge Taylor & Francis Group, pp. 51–80.

11. Holt JB (2007) The topography of poverty in the United States: A spatial analysis using county-level data from the community health status indicators project. Preventing Chronic Disease: Public Health Research, Practice, and Policy, http://cdc.gov/pcd/issues/2007/oct/07_0091.htm.

12. Murray CJL, Kulkarni S, Ezzati M (2005) Eight Americas: New perspectives on U.S. health disparities. Am J Prev Med 29: 4–10.

13. Hotez PJ (2012) Tropical diseases: The new plague of poverty. New York Times, August 18.

14. Parise ME, Hotez PJ, Slutsker L (2014) Neglected parasitic infections in the United States: Needs and opportunities. Am J Trop Med Hyg 90(5): 783–85.

15. Hotez PJ, Wilkins PP (2009) Toxocariasis: America's most common neglected infection of poverty and a helminthiasis of global importance? PLOS Negl Trop Dis 3(3): e400.

16. Won KY, Kruzon-Moran D, Schantz PM, Jones JL (2008) National seroprevalence and risk factors for zoonotic Toxocara spp. infection. Am J Trop Med Hyg 79(4): 552–57.

17. Walsh MG, Haseeb MA (2014) Toxocariasis and lung function: Relevance of a neglected infection in an urban landscape. Acta Parasitol 59(1): 126–31.

18. Walsh MG, Haseeb MA (2012) Reduced cognitive function in children with toxocariasis in a nationally representative sample of the United States. Int J Parasitol 42(13–14):1159–63.

19. Hotez PJ (2014) Neglected infections of poverty in the United States and their effects on the brain. JAMA Psychiatry 71(10): 1099–100.

20. Lee RM, Moore LB, Bottazzi ME, Hotez PJ (2014) Toxocariasis in North America: A systematic review. PLOS Negl Trop Dis 8(8): e3116.

21. Garcia HH, Nash TE, Del Brutoo OH (2014) Clinical symptoms, diagnosis, and treatment of neurocysticercosis. Lancet Neurol 13(12): 1202–15.

22. Bern C, Kjos S, Yabsley MJ, Montgomery SP (2011) Trypanosoma cruzi and Chagas disease in the United States. Clin Microbiol Rev 24(4): 655–81.

23. Garcia MN, Aguilar D, Gorchakov R, Rossmann SN, Montgomery SP, Rivera H, Woc-Colburn L, Hotez PJ, Murray KO (2015) Evidence of autochthonous Chagas disease in southeastern Texas. Am J Trop Med Hyg 92(2): 325–30.

24. Garcia MN, Murray KO, Hotez PJ, Rossmann SN, Gorchakov R, Ontiveros A, Woc-Colburn L, et al. (2015) Development of Chagas cardiac manifestations among Texas blood donors. Am J Cardiol 115(1): 113–17.

25. Garcia MN, Woc-Colburn L, Rossmann SN, Townsend RL, Stramer SL, Bravo M, Kamel H, et al. (2014) Trypanosoma cruzi screening in Texas blood donors, 2008–12. Epidemiol Infect [Epub ahead of print].

26. Garcia MN, Hotez PJ, Murray KO (2014) Potential novel risk factors for autochthonous and sylvatic transmission of human Chagas disease in the United States. Parasites Vectors 7: 311.

27. Tenney TD, Curtis-Robles R, Snowden KF, Hamer SA (2014) Shelter dogs as sentinels for Trypanosoma cruzi transmission across Texas. Emerg Infect Dis 20(8): 1323–26.

28. Andrus J, Bottazzi ME, Chow J, Goraleski KA, Fisher-Hoch SP, Lambuth JK, Lee BY, et al. (2013) Ears of the armadillo: Global health research and neglected diseases in Texas. PLOS Negl Trop Dis 7(6): e2021.

29. Jones JL, Kruszon-Moran D, Won K, Wilson M, Schantz PM (2008) Toxoplasma gondii and Toxocara spp. co-infection. Am J Trop Med Hyg 78(1): 35–39.

30. Jones JL, Kruszon-Moran D, Rivera HN, Price C, Wilkins PP (2014) Toxoplasma gondii seroprevalence in the United States 2009–2010 and comparsion with the past two decades. Am J Trop Med Hyg 90(6): 1135–39.

31. Jones JL, Parise ME, Fiore AE (2014) Neglected parasitic infections in the United States: Toxoplasmosis. Am J Trop Med Hyg 90(5): 794–99.

32. Torrey EF, Yolken RH (2014) The urban risk and migration risk factors for schizophrenia: Are cats the answer? Schizophr Res 159(2–3): 299–302.

33. Coleman JS, Gaydos CA, Witter F (2013) Trichomonas vaginalis vaginitis in obstetrics and gynecology practice: New concepts and controversies. Obstet Gynecol Surv 68(1): 43–50.

34. Meites E (2013) Trichomoniasis: The "neglected" sexually transmitted disease. Infect Dis Clin North Am 27(4): 755–64.

35. Sutton M, Sternberg M, Koumans EH, McQuillan G, Berman S, et al (2007) The prevalence of Trichomonas vaginalis infection among reproductive-age women in the United States, 2001–2004. Clin Infect Dis 45: 1319–26.

36. Kissinger P, Amedee A, Clark RA, Dumestre J, Theall KP, et al (2009) Trichomonas vaginalis treatment reduces vaginal HIV-1 shedding. Sex Transm Dis 36: 11–16.

37. Quinlivan EB, Patel SN, Gordensky CA, Golin CE, Tien HC, et al. (2012) Modeling the impact of Trichomonas vaginalis infection on HIV transmission in HIV-infected individuals in medical care. Sex Transm Dis 39: 671–77.

38. Kraemer MU, Sinka ME, Duda KA, Mylne AQ, Shearer FM, Barker CM, Moore CG, et al. (2015) The global distribution of the arbovirus vectors Aedes aegypti and Ae. albopictus. Elife 4: doi: 10.7554/eLife.08347.

39. Hotez PJ, Murray KO, Buekens P (2014) The Gulf Coast: A new American underbelly of tropical diseases and poverty. PLOS Negl Trop Dis 8(5): e2760.

40. Murray KO, Rodriguez LF, Herrington E, Kharat V, Vasilakis N, Walker C, Turner C, et al. (2013) Identification of dengue fever cases in Houston, Texas, with evidence of autochthonous transmission between 2003 and 2005. Vector Borne Zoonotic Dis 13(12): 835–45.

41. Garcia MN, Hasbun R, Murray KO (2015) Persistence of West Nile virus. Microbes Infect 17(2): 163–68.

42. Weatherhead JE, Miller VE, Garcia MN, Hasbun R, Salazar L, Dimachkie MM, Murray KO (2015) Long-term neurological outcomes in West Nile virus–infected patients: An observational study. Am J Trop Med Hyg 92(5): 1006–12.

43. Murray KO, Ruktanonchai D, Hesalroad D, Fonken E, Nolan MS (2013) West Nile virus, Texas, USA, 2012. Emerg Infect Dis 19(11): 1836–38.

44. Nolan MS, Podoll AS, Hause AM, Akers KM, Finkel KW, Murray KO (2012) Prevalence of chronic kidney disease and progression of disease over time among patients enrolled in the Houston West Nile virus cohort. PLOS One 7(7): e40374.

45. Nolan MS, Hause AM, Murray KO (2012) Findings of long-term depression up to 8 years post infection from West Nile virus. J Clin Psychol 68(7): 801–8.

46. Montgomery RR, Murray KO (2015) Risk factors for West Nile virus infection and disease in populations and individuals. Expert Rev Anti Infect Ther 13(3): 317–25.

47. Meyer TE, Bull LM, Cain Holmes K, Pascua RF, Travassos da Rosa A, Gutierrez CR, Corbin T, et al. (2007) West Nile infection among the homeless, Houston. Emerg Infect Dis 13(10): 1500–1503.

48. http://www.cdc.gov/hiv/group/racialethnic/africanamericans/index.html.

49. Maulsby C, Millett G, Lindsey K, Kelley R, Johnson K, Montoya D, Holtgrave D (2014) HIV among black men who have sex with men (MSM) in the United States: A review of the literature. AIDS Behav 18(1): 10–25.

50. Shrage L (2015) Why Are So Many Black Women Dying of AIDS? New York Times, December 11, http://www.nytimes.com/2015/12/12/opinion/why-are-so-many -black-women-dying-of-aids.html?_r=0.

51. http://www.cdc.gov/tb/topic/populations/default.htm.

52. http://www.cdc.gov/tb/topic/populations/HealthDisparities/default.htm.

53. http://www.cdc.gov/tb/topic/populations/homelessness/default.htm.

54. Stimpert KK, Montgomery SP (2010) Physician awareness of Chagas disease, USA. Emerg Infect Dis 16(5): 871–72.

55. Verani JR, Montgomery SP, Schulkin J, Anderson B, Jones JL (2010) Survey of obstetrician-gynecologists in the United States about Chagas disease. Am J Trop Med Hyg 83(4): 891–95.

56. http://openstates.org/tx/bills/84/HB2055.

57. https://www.govtrack.us/congress/bills/114/hr2897/text.

58. https://www.govtrack.us/congress/bills/114/hr1797.

59. https://www.congress.gov/bill/114th-congress/house-bill/6.

60. Bilbe G (2015) Infectious diseases: Overcoming neglect of kinetoplastid diseases. Science 348(6238): 974–76.

61. Dumonteil E, Bottazzi ME, Zhan B, Heffernan MJ, Jones K, Valenzuela JG, Kamhawi S, et al. (2012) Accelerating the development of a therapeutic vaccine for human Chagas disease: Rationale and prospects. Expert Rev Vaccines 11(9): 1043–55.

Chapter 11. The G20

1. Rawls J ([1971] 1999) A Theory of Justice, rev. ed. Cambridge, MA: Belknap Press, p. 13.

2. Hotez PJ (2015) Blue marble health redux: Neglected tropical diseases and human development in the Group of 20 (G20) nations and Nigeria. PLOS Negl Trop Dis 9(8): e0004035.

3. http://www.who.int/neglected_diseases/preventive_chemotherapy/sth/en.

4. http://www.who.int/neglected_diseases/preventive_chemotherapy/sch/en.

5. http://www.who.int/neglected_diseases/preventive_chemotherapy/lf/en.

6. http://policycures.org/gfinder.html.

7. https://www.ghitfund.org/hww/businessmodel.

8. Slingsby BT, Kurokawa K (2013) The Global Health Innovative Technology (GHIT) Fund: Financing medical innovations for neglected populations. Lancet Glob Health 1(4): e184–85.

9. http://www.nytimes.com/interactive/2015/07/24/business/international/the -world-according-to-china-investment-maps.html?hp&action=click&pgtype=Home page&module=photo-spot-region&region=top-news&WT.nav=top-news.

10. http://policycures.org/downloads/GF_GermanReport_English.pdf.

11. Von Philipsborn P, Steinbeis F, Bender ME, Regmi S, Tinnemann P (2015) Poverty-related and neglected diseases—an economic and epidemiological analysis of poverty relatedness and neglect in research and development. Global Health Action 8: 25818.

12. http://ec.europa.eu/research/fp7/index_en.cfm.

13. http://hookvac.eu.

14. http://ec.europa.eu/programmes/horizon2020/en/what-horizon-2020.

15. http://www.edctp.org.

16. https://g20.org.

17. https://g20.org/wp-content/uploads/2014/12/2015-TURKEY-G-20-PRESI DENCY-FINAL.pdf.

18. http://nam.edu/perspectives-2013-strengthening-mechanisms-to-prioritize -coordinate-finance-and-execute-rd-to-meet-health-needs-in-developing-countries.

19. Plotkin SA, Mahmoud AAF, Farrar J (2015) Establishing a global vaccine-development fund. N Engl J Med 373: 297–99.

20. Balasegaram M, Bréchot C, Farrar J, Heymann D, Ganguly N, Khor M, et al. (2015) A global biomedical R&D fund and mechanism for innovations of public health importance. PLOS Med 12(5): e1001831.

21. http://www.who.int/research-observatory/publications/ro_whadoc/en.

22. http://www.who.int/tdr/news/2015/tdr_manage_pooled_RnD_fund/en.

23. Hotez P, Singh SK, Zhou X-N (2013) Advancing Sino-Indian cooperation to combat tropical diseases. PLOS Negl Trop Dis 7(9): e2204.

24. http://bakerinstitute.org/research/ blue-marble-health-new-presidential-roadmap-global-poverty-related-diseases.

25. http://www.wipo.int/research/en.

26. Hotez PJ (2014) Global Christianity and the control of its neglected tropical diseases. PLOS Negl Trop Dis 8(11): e3135.

Chapter 12. A Framework for Science and Vaccine Diplomacy

1. Hotez PJ (2010) Nuclear weapons and neglected diseases: The "ten-thousand-to-one Gap." PLOS Negl Trop Dis 4(4): e680.

2. Hotez P, Singh SK, Zhou X-N (2013) Advancing Sino-Indian cooperation to combat tropical diseases. PLOS Negl Trop Dis 7(9): e2204.

3. Hotez PJ (2014) "Vaccine diplomacy": Historical perspectives and future directions. PLOS Negl Trop Dis 8(6): e2808.

4. http://www.who.int/topics/international_health_regulations/en.

5. Maurice J (2015) Expert panel slams WHO's poor showing against Ebola. Lancet 386(9990): e1.

6. Gostin LO, DeBartolo M, Friedman EA (2015) The international health regulations 10 years on: The governing framework for global health security. Lancet 386: 2222–26.

7. http://www.globalhealth.gov/global-health-topics/global-health-security/ghs agenda.html.

8. Jamison DT, Summers LH, Alleyne G, Arrow S, Berkley S, et al. (2013) Global health 2035: A world converging within a generation. Lancet 382(9908): 1898–955.

9. http://www.worldbank.org/en/topic/health/brief/global-financing-facility-in -support-of-every-woman-every-child.

10. Hotez PJ (2009) The neglected tropical diseases and their devastating health and economic impact on the member nations of the Organisation of the Islamic Conference. PLOS Negl Trop Dis 3(10): e539.

11. Hotez PJ, Herricks J (2015) Impact of the neglected tropical diseases on human development in the Organisation of Islamic Cooperation Nations. PLOS Negl Trop Dis 9(11): e0003782; doi:10.1371/journal.pntd.0003782.

12. http://tamest.org/blog/entry/my-activities-as-united-states-science-envoy.

13. https://www.whitehouse.gov/the-press-office/remarks-president-cairo-uni versity-6-04-09.

14. Hotez PJ (2015) Vaccine science diplomacy: Expanding capacity to prevent emerging and neglected tropical diseases arising from Islamic State (IS)–held territories. PLOS Negl Trop Dis 9(9): e0003852; doi:10.1371/journal.pntd.0003852.

15. Hotez PJ (2015) Combating the next lethal epidemic. Science 348: 296–97.

16. Hotez PJ, Bottazzi ME, Strych U (2016) New vaccines for the world's poorest people. Ann Rev Med 67 (January): 405–17.

Chapter 13. Future Directions

1. GBD 2013 Mortality and Causes of Death Collaborators (2015) Global, regional, and national age-sex specific all-cause and cause-specific mortality for 240 causes of death, 1990–2013: A systematic analysis for the Global Burden of Disease Study 2013. Lancet 385: 117–71.

2. Global Burden of Disease Study 2013 Collaborators (2015) Global, regional, and national incidence, prevalence, and years lived with disability for 301 acute and chronic diseases and injuries in 188 countries, 1990-2013: a systematic analysis for the Global Burden of Disease Study 2013. Lancet 386: 743–800.

3. http://www.who.int/bulletin/volumes/92/9/14–020914/en.

4. Hotez PJ (2011) New antipoverty drugs, vaccines, and diagnostics: A research agenda for the US President's Global Health Initiative (GHI). PLOS Negl Trop Dis 5(5): e1133.

5. WHO (2015) Planning, requesting medicines and reporting for preventive chemotherapy. Weekly Epidemiol Rec 90(14): 133–48.

6. http://www.dcvmn.org/-About-.

7. http://www.who.int/immunization/research/committees/pdvac/en.

Index

About the Author

Peter J. Hotez, MD, PhD, is dean of the National School of Tropical Medicine and Professor of Pediatrics and Molecular Virology & Microbiology at Baylor College of Medicine, where he is also the Texas Children's Hospital Endowed Chair of Tropical Pediatrics. He is the president of the Sabin Vaccine Institute and the Fellow in Disease and Poverty at the James A. Baker III Institute for Public Policy at Rice University, as well as University Professor in Biology at Baylor University.

Dr. Hotez is an internationally recognized physician-scientist in neglected tropical diseases and vaccine development. He leads the only product development partnership for developing new vaccines for hookworm infection, schistosomiasis, Chagas disease, and SARS/MERS—diseases that affect hundreds of millions of children and adults worldwide. In 2006 at the Clinton Global Initiative, he cofounded the Global Network for Neglected Tropical Diseases to provide access to essential medicines for hundreds of millions of people.

Dr. Hotez has authored more than four hundred original scientific articles and is the author of *Forgotten People, Forgotten Diseases*. He is an elected member of the National Academy of Medicine (formerly the Institute of Medicine), and in 2011, he was awarded the Abraham Horwitz Award for Excellence in Leadership in Inter-American Public Health by the Pan American Health Organization of the World Health Organization. In 2014, the White House and US State Department selected Dr. Hotez as a United States science envoy.